Radiant Health & Happiness is Possible

How I Healed From Chronic Fatigue Syndrome

MARGO NAGY

ISBN:0615538789
ISBN-13:9780615538785

CONTENTS

~   Introduction   1

I   My Journey   4

II   Chronic Reversed Polarity   35

III   Unconscious Emotions & Beliefs   40

IV   Stress   58

V   Energy Healing   78

VI   Eating Optimally   89

VII   Loving Yourself   93

VIII   Connecting to God & Your Higher Self   99

IX   The Power of Your Mind   106

~   The Keys to Achieving Health & Happiness   112

~   Resources   114

~   About the Author   116

~   More Exercises   118

DEDICATION

I dedicate this book to my mom and Master Herbalist Keith Smith. Until I met Keith Smith, my mom is the only one who understood me and was always there for me when I was sick for so long. I am so grateful for her unconditional love and support. And if I hadn't met Keith Smith who discovered "Chronic Reversed Polarity", I wouldn't be here writing this book! Thank you Keith for this amazing discovery, your Herbal Program, and your sincere understanding and support.

INTRODUCTION

Are You Ready to Heal?

This may seem like a silly question, but you would be surprised at how many people are not ready to heal, and that is okay. So ask yourself right now, "Am I ready to heal?" If you are not ready, then ask yourself why. Maybe you are scared? Maybe you don't believe it is possible? Or maybe you are not ready to be on your mission, your soul's purpose on this planet? I sensed that I had a big mission of writing this book and traveling the world helping people. This was overwhelming at times especially when I was tired and so used to being sick and sort of "hiding out" for so many years. Don't worry if you don't have a big mission, or you don't know what your mission is. Many of us are here to spread love and light, and that can be done as easily as smiling at a stranger as they pass by.

If you aren't ready to heal, but want to be, then ask God and the angels to help you. You know the old saying, "You can lead a horse to water…but you can't make them drink." Well that is true, especially with healing.

Do you believe that you can heal and totally recover? This is also extremely important for healing to occur. What we believe is what we attract, and so if you do believe that you can heal, then you will. If you don't, or are not sure yet...then please read on with an open mind and heart and ask for help from God and the angels if you desire.

Now that you are ready to heal...come with me on this magical journey of healing. I ask that you read this book with an open mind. Some concepts may be new or foreign to you. To be able to fully embrace them and understand them, you also need to be willing to change. I was willing to try everything and do anything in order to heal...and it has finally paid off. Now I can help others heal themselves by normalizing their polarity so they don't have to try everything else. I have 26 years of experience with Chronic Fatigue Syndrome/CFS, depression, other illnesses and the healing process. I know that I went through all of the pain and suffering and ultimate relief/healing in order to help others. In fact that is precisely what kept me going and not giving up. I am living proof that you CAN heal from CFS and depression.

In this book, I share my journey of being on the Alpine Ski Team at University of Colorado, Boulder when I was 19, to being bed ridden for months, to almost dying. For 26 years I struggled with Chronic Fatigue Syndrome and other illness. I battled intense fatigue and weakness, coped with constant disappointment and depression, and tried absolutely everything possible to recover. Using conventional western medicine and alternative healing methods gave me extensive experience of the healing process. Attending the School of Energy Mastery revealed the power of energy healing and the importance of healing the emotional and mental body along with the physical body. However, after healing again and again only to relapse over and over, I finally discovered Chronic Reversed Polarity, the key to incurable diseases thanks to Keith Smith, Master Herbalist.

Un-reversing my polarity is what healed me permanently. This is explained along with other valuable tools to healing. In this book I give support, guidance, resources, empowerment, first hand experience, compassion, relief, a shift in consciousness, inspiration, hope and most importantly understanding. As you know, if you are suffering from CFS…no-one understands unless they have personally experienced it. So hang in there…because you CAN heal from CFS, depression and other illnesses and conditions. **Radiant health and happiness…is possible!**

* * *

I

MY JOURNEY

My journey starts in Montclair, California, August 22, 1963. I come into this world a Leo, with grandiose dreams and burning determination. Here I am, the youngest of seven including two deaf sisters, and one deaf brother. My mother, busy taking care of everyone, and overwhelmed at times, manages to spend time with me. Most of my brothers and sisters are much older than me and are already out of the house. My brother Ted, who is just a few years older than me, is off to a boarding school for the deaf in St. Louis for most of the year. So...my mom and I have time to go to the zoo and do fun things like that. My father on the other hand is very busy providing for such a big family, which he does very well. However, I'm perceiving this as... not getting enough attention. After all, I'm a Leo and we love attention!

I am so fortunate to have the opportunity do whatever I desire. We go skiing in the winters and water skiing in the summers. I play all sports and take ballet lessons and piano lessons. My world abounds with unlimited possibilities. I actually think money grows on trees. This part of my life is very much like a fairytale.

A few years after I am born, my dad becomes an alcoholic. Like so many families, ours is dysfunctional. Of course, I always wonder…is there really such a thing as a "normal" family? Because of the alcoholism, I become codependent. I start to feel responsible for others happiness. I want to take care of others, and unconsciously, put others needs before mine. I really just want everyone to be happy. My extreme sensitivity allows me to pretty much feel everything that is going on around me and within other people. So even though people aren't saying how they really feel or if they feel anything…I'm knowing exactly how everyone is feeling, and trying my hardest to keep the peace and make everyone happy. I don't realize until much later, that this can be extremely draining!

My father is very competitive, which rubs off on me. He had been an alternate swimmer for the 1932 Olympics. Throughout his life, he continues to race in the Masters Swim Program and The Dolphin Club in the San Francisco Bay. In order to get his attention, I become an over-achiever. I strive to be the best at everything and being anything less is unacceptable. I put so much stress on myself trying to achieve all of this. "Not feeling good enough," definitely originates here. If I don't win an athletic event it doesn't seem to matter, or be good enough for my Dad's approval. At least that's the way I am interpreting it, which, unfortunately…will stay with me most of my life.

My competitive life starts in grade school where I play all the sports and am most valuable player on the softball team and basketball team. At 14, I start playing tennis. We actually move to a country club that has 10 tennis courts with lights. I'm in heaven, I get to play tennis for four hours every day, and play in tennis tournaments on weekends. My dream is to play in Wimbledon someday. My private coach says that I am good enough to go to Stanford on a tennis scholarship. I also want to go to a tennis academy in Southern California, but my mom doesn't want me to leave home. After three deaf brothers and sisters have gone away to a boarding school for the deaf in St. Louis from an early age to the 8th grade, I don't think she wants me to leave home yet.

It's now my junior year in high school, I'm so unhappy with my home life, I start partying. I'm also really frustrated because there are not any good female tennis players to practice with, so I start ski racing instead. I started skiing when I was 4 years old, but I'm just starting to race at 16. This begins on the Ski Team at Alpine Meadows Ski Resort in Lake Tahoe, CA.

My Polarity Becomes Reversed

It's still my junior year and I'm on my way skiing with a friend. I just got a used Mustang and I'm so exited to go on a ski trip. It's raining hard and my Dad really doesn't want me to go. However, because I am so spoiled and head strong...I go anyway.

We are about an hour from the ski resort and it is dark already. There is a leak in my power steering, which I already know about and haven't fixed yet...so I stop to fill it up before we head up the mountain. 30 minutes later, we are driving on a windy mountain road and it is pouring down rain, when the power steering goes out. We are headed towards a tight turn and the steering wheel is not functioning properly. I shout to my friend, "It's not turning!" We go straight off the road and hit a tree going about 50 miles an hour! As I open my eyes and look around in total shock...I feel God right next to me and it feels like he's saying that I almost died, but he's giving me another chance. Luckily we were driving a Mustang II that had a long front end, otherwise we could have been killed. I bent the steering wheel with my head and suffered a mild concussion, temporary amnesia, along with some cuts on my face. Fortunately my friend is not seriously injured either. However, this is probably when my polarity becomes reversed. My life drastically changes after this. At this point I don't know about "Chronic Reversed Polarity" (further explained in Chapter II) and how it keeps your body from functioning normally.

In the process of trying to be on the U.S. Ski Team, I begin abusing my body and over doing it. After high school, I attend Ski Etude Race Academy in Incline Village, Lake Tahoe, where the Epstein Barr Virus was first diagnosed. In the early 1980's, 250 people in that small town are diagnosed with this virus. Now I'm 18 years old, and I think I'm superwoman! I go to parties and bars, party until 2am, then get up at 8:00am and go to aerobics or ski train. I don't party every night, but definitely burn the candle at both ends. Completely unaware that I am hypoglycemic and shouldn't be drinking alcohol or eating sugar, I think everyone gets as hung-over as I do.

One day on the race course, my arm gets caught on a gate and my shoulder is dislocated. A doctor in Incline Village does laser surgery, "Arthroscopy" on my shoulder. This is the first surgery I have. Surgeries can also reverse your polarity. Then my other shoulder gets dislocated several times, it becomes globally instable… so they put a screw in it. Fortunately, it worked!

After one year in Lake Tahoe, I attend school at the University of Colorado in Boulder. I'm on the Alpine Ski Team, and enrolled in the School of Engineering, to be an architect. Again I think I am superwoman. I enroll in five extremely hard courses, train extensively every day, and travel to races. After only one year, my father loses a lot of money in the stock market and can't afford to pay for my out of state tuition anymore. I'm devastated! The stress of not having money and not being able to pursue my dream of being on the US Ski Team causes me to succumb to the Epstein Barr Virus and Chronic Fatigue Syndrome/CFS. Because my polarity has been reversed since the car accident, my immune system is compromised leaving me unable to fight off invasive and harmful viruses, illnesses, and diseases. I don't want to move back to California and stop skiing. So I move to Vail, Colorado to be a ski instructor in hopes of attaining in state residency in order to continue my education and ski racing at Boulder.

Chronic Fatigue Syndrome Starts

This is when I start getting sick. The stress of not having money and not being able to do what I want to do is intense. I have been so used to having whatever I wanted growing up...yes, I am spoiled. I also haven't learned to appreciate the value of money. Not having money is a real shock. In many ways my dreams are shattered. Being on the Ski Team at C.U. is the stepping stone to being on the U.S. Ski Team one day. Now that dream will be harder to attain.

Teaching skiing in Vail is great fun. Again, I start partying and pushing myself physically by skiing all day everyday. After ski school, we hit the "Après-Ski" bars, eat free hors d'oeuvres, and drink like fishes. No wonder I am getting dizzy on the chairlift and almost fainting while standing in line for lunch! Seriously, I am getting dizzy on the chairlift and while waiting in line at lunch I feel faint. During my childhood, I had fainted several times when I hadn't eaten in 4-5 hours. However, my family doctor said it was just part of my growing. Doctors do not acknowledge my Hypoglycemia.

This is when my incredibly frustrating visits to the doctors start. In Denver, I see an internist who gives me a glucose tolerance test. After nearly fainting and passing out in the waiting room several times, he says I'm only "borderline" hypoglycemic! He says that I am just an athlete who is in tune with my body. However, I read a book about hypoglycemia and know deep down that I have it. Unfortunately, those six hour glucose tolerance tests are not accurate.

While I'm training gates one day in Vail, the ski coach from Colorado Mountain College in Leadville recruits me to be on his ski team. At first I'm not that excited because it isn't C.U. (a major University with one of the best ski teams), but it is a free ride and free skiing. The school is in Leadville, Colorado, which is 10,000 feet above sea level. It is an old, almost deserted mining town, so there isn't much to do except study and ski. I get straight A's, stop partying, and eat healthy. However, my health is still rapidly deteriorating.

Its a few days before my first race of the year, and I am sick with bronchitis, which I have gotten faithfully every year since I was a young child. Even though I am on antibiotics, I don't want to miss the first race in Aspen. So I go to the week long training camp and race with a temperature. The first collegiate race of the season is on the last day. Even though I'm sick, I want to race anyway. I am so weak I barely make it through the race course and collapse at the finish line.

Before the next race in Utah, I come down with Pelvic Inflammatory Disease. Unfortunately, this is so acute I can't go to Utah. The morning we are supposed to leave, I am rushed to the emergency room. I finish the ski season and attend more races; although, I keep getting sick or injured. At the end of the year, I graduate from Colorado Mountain College with an AA. After such a disappointing ski season and deteriorating health, I have no choice but to stop ski racing. My dream of being on the US Ski Team is officially over.

Now I'm moving back to California to get my BA degree in Business. Because of my ill health and inability to attend school full-time or work and attend school at the same time, I attend four more colleges. Being "reversed" and suffering from Chronic Fatigue Syndrome/CFS is greatly affecting my mind. In school, I can barely concentrate. I'm always in a fog. My attention span is extremely limited and my memory is horrible, basically non-existent at times. One time, at the checkout register in a grocery store, I could not remember my phone number. Sometimes I can barely recall my address or zip code!

I'm attending school in California now, and my health is deteriorating further. Not only am I not skiing anymore, I am not able to do any sports or exercise. I go to the gym occasionally, and I become weak and dizzy after only 10 minutes. I moved back to Southern California to attend California State Polytechnic University in Pomona. It is so smoggy! When I first moved in September, I couldn't see any mountains. Now…a couple of months later, in the winter when the smog has cleared… there is a mountain range right in front of me! This is when I realize how smoggy it is. Smog is bad for your health especially when you are already sick.

To get away from the smog, I move to Newport Beach, which is still smoggy, but not as bad because it is along the ocean. I work part-time and go to school part-time. At work I am pretty "out of it" most of the time and always light-headed. However, I start racing once a week for the ski team at the ski shop where I work. This is fun, until I get really weak and dizzy on the chairlift. Completely exhausted, I can only ski a few runs. Then I can barely finish the race course. At the end of the day, I look and feel like a rag doll that has just completed a marathon. Many times on the 3 hour drive back home from the ski area... I feel sick. I'm trying to use "mind over matter" and pretend that I don't have CFS - but it is not working. I also go out dancing occasionally, and then I am completely bed ridden and wiped out for a couple of days.

For a while I live with my boyfriend that I met in Vail. He did not know me before I had CFS, so he just assumes I am "lazy" because I am so tired all the time. Luckily my best friend from high school comes to visit me. She can see that something is wrong with me, and that it isn't all in my head. She remembers me being an enthusiastic person and having so much energy in high school. After this, I leave my boyfriend and move in with my parents for a while to go to doctors. I am so sick and weak that I can't even drive. On the way to a doctor appointment, while driving across the Bay Bridge into San Francisco, I become panicky. Just driving into the city stresses my body so much I can barely handle it - even though my mother is driving. A doctor in San Francisco takes blood tests and finds that the Epstein Barr Virus is active. Finally, a doctor acknowledges that it's not "all in my head"...unfortunately, he is unable to cure it. It is so frustrating trying to get people, family and friends to understand. My father looks at me and says, "Gee honey, you are the best looking sick person I've ever seen." He is implying that I couldn't possibly be that sick, right? Heck, I don't look it!

Because I am so sick, and my polarity is reversed, I become really depressed. I go to a therapist and even she doesn't understand. She is treating me as if I am just depressed. People don't understand that I am depressed because I am sick and too weak to do the things I love, like play tennis and go skiing. Also I am not able to be who I really am capable of being! I'm not meeting my own expectations at all and it is so frustrating and depressing. I have such big ambitions and goals that are unattainable. For example, I want to be a business executive, run my own company, and make lots of money. My therapist says, "Just put your tennis shoes by your bed, and as soon as you get up in the morning... go for a walk." Well, helloooo! If I had the energy to get up and out of bed and actually go for a walk in the morning... I wouldn't be so depressed!!!

At 23, I'm going to an acupuncturist who is very helpful. He confirms my hypoglycemia and warns me that if I continue to drink alcohol, I will become diabetic and need to give myself insulin shots. Well… that is enough for me to stop drinking… thank God! So I stop drinking, and I start to be more aware of my diet, especially my sugar intake. I always have snacks with me and try to eat something every 2-3 hours to keep my blood sugar stabilized. This helps greatly.

I am living with my mom and dad now which I haven't done for ten years. I am working part time at a tennis club and seeing doctors. At work I get a call…my dad has died of a heart attack while trying to break the record for 80 year olds in a Masters Swim Race! My father competed until the day he died. This is so hard on my mother. She has always been so strong emotionally and now she is really depressed without my dad. My dad stopped drinking a few years ago and has been so sweet and loving. We are both so depressed it is really hard living here. So I am moving back to Newport Beach.

After working in a ski shop for a couple of years while going to school, I start driving limousines. The money is good, but the hours are horrendous. I stop going to school for a while and drive limo's full time. Some days I work 12-20 hours. Of course, a lot of that time I am just waiting around, but it is still work. Sometimes I only get 4 hours of sleep. Driving on the freeways between Los Angeles to San Diego is also not the healthiest work environment. Occasionally, I drive from Newport Beach to LAX twice a day. The area within an hour from LAX is extremely smoggy and again, my health is seriously deteriorating. I occasionally drink caffeine and eat junk food, which is really detrimental to my body.

Then I start taking "pep" pills from the health food store. They claim to be caffeine-free and be a "natural" energizer. However, they contain Majuang a stimulant that completely taxes my adrenals and nervous system. I am pushing myself too hard, working long hours and taking pep pills.

Lowest Point in my Healing Journey

One morning, I wake up and have a terrible stomach ache. I'm in the bathroom on the toilet, experiencing diarrhea. The pain in my stomach is so intense I become really dizzy and faint. Next thing I know, I am laying on the bathroom floor coming in and out of consciousness. I am trembling and sweating and lose control of my bodily functions. It is extremely scary. At this point… I think I'm dying! I'm staying at a friend's house who is out of town on business. I am alone, so I call my mother. She lives too far away to do anything. So I call a nutritionist I am seeing. She has seen this coming on and has been asking me several times, "When are you going to go away somewhere out of the smog and stress to rest and take care of yourself?" She says, "Are you ready to follow my advice now?" Yes, I am ready! I am so weak, I can't even drive. So I leave my car in Southern California and have a friend drive me to my mom's house in Northern California, eight hours away.

I spend one year with my brother Mark who lives in the foothills of Northern California. I am very fortunate to have a place to stay out in the country with clean air. This is the lowest point of my illness. I am in bed for three months. I can't even go grocery shopping for about a month. When I go for a walk I can barely walk across the street. My brother lives near a country road where cars drive really fast. I am so incredibly weak… I am afraid I will fall walking across the road and get hit by a car! My insomnia is so bad, I can't fall asleep until around 4:00 am some nights. Then I sleep for 12 hours. Sometimes I'm so tired, I feel like I am paralyzed – this is scary. I sleep a lot during the day, watch movies and TV. I think I've seen every movie ever made. Unfortunately, I am so out of it, I can't read. Late at night, I lie in bed and daydream about what I will do when I get better. Fortunately, I haven't "given up" yet. My eyes tear thinking about how sad, frustrated, and lonely I am.

After three months of resting, and taking supplements, I feel good enough to attend school. So I go to California State University, Sacramento for one year. It is nice having a place to live free of rent, so I can just go to school, study and rest. During Christmas break, which lasts a month, I'm trying out to be a ski instructor at Squaw Valley Ski Resort in Lake Tahoe California. Even though I'm out of shape and I haven't skied in a long time, I am chosen. For making the cut, I receive a free lift ticket to ski the next day. Unfortunately, I am so wiped out from just trying out… I wonder if I even have the strength and stamina to actually be a ski instructor. Sure enough, the next day I am in my car in the parking lot. I am so exhausted, I don't know if I have enough energy to ski. So I put my ski pants on and am even more tired just doing that! Here I am sitting in my car with a free lift ticket valued at $50. I look up at the ski area, and just cry. I am too tired to ski, and definitely not well enough to be a ski instructor. I have to quit before I even start.

Health Improves a Little

After a year at my brother's, I move back to Newport Beach, and I get a job at Newport Beach Tennis Club. I like being in the tennis environment again, but it is very frustrating working here because I am still too sick to play much tennis. I am so out of shape and weak that I can only play once every week or two, and only play for about ten to twenty minutes. When I play, I get really light-headed and dizzy and am wiped out the next day or two.

One night after work, I play tennis with a young girl who is a really good tennis player. I know I should only play for about twenty minutes, but I am having so much fun I can't stop. Its night time and we are playing on center court, under the lights with bleachers all around us. I can hear the echo of the ball being hit, which is a really amazing sound and feeling. It amplifies everything you are doing and you feel like a real pro! I am in heaven playing with such a good tennis player. After about 45 minutes, I am so out of it - I twist my ankle going for a volley and break it! I have never broken a bone before.

After my ankle heals, I start skiing again occasionally. I can't ski for very long, but the clean air in the mountains makes me feel so much better. Unfortunately, my body can't really handle the skiing. Getting dizzy and lightheaded on the chairlift is scary because I don't want to faint and fall off the chairlift and plunge hundreds of feet.

In May of 1993 while I am skiing in Mammoth, CA, I meet Alex. My sister Marianna is dying of cancer at the age of 41. I am really sad and vulnerable. When I meet Alex, it is love at first sight. The first night we meet, we talk for hours about CFS, health and vitamins. He knows so much about vitamins. I am so excited that I don't scare him away with my illness. I don't realize he has an "illness" of his own… he is a drug addict. He is so athletic and successful, and is the top salesman for solar in California. I have no idea he is an addict.

In the beginning, he is so full of life and passion. We go on many ski trips and surf trips together. His vitality and zest rub off on me and truly lift my spirits. We have so much fun, although most of the time, he is smoking pot or using cocaine and drinking. The more time I spend with him, the more I realize how much he parties. At first it was hard to tell, because he was so functional while being "stoned." I am also so in love with him and in love with the kind of life we live, I don't see what is really going on with him

Now I'm in school again getting closer to graduating. Unfortunately, every time I change schools, it sets me back a semester or two. My health improves during the first six months we are together because of all the love and good feelings. He also helps me eat very healthy. Six months after we meet we move in together. Being a part of his daily life and being more involved in his crazy life becomes very stressful for me. We get married six months later in 1994. I am not happy because he is gone most of the time working and surfing and God only knows what else! I am also extremely frustrated with my health. I am able to attend school full time, but I'm not healthy enough to workout and physically get back into shape, which makes it hard to physically keep up with Alex. I try not to party because it is so detrimental to my health. However, I do occasionally. Then I'm sick, weak and depressed for days or weeks. I definitely can't lead the kind of lifestyle he is leading. He uses cocaine occasionally and comes home all drugged out.

This is really disappointing and stressful for me. A couple of times I go to a hotel to get away. I can't be around him when he is doing this. I definitely can't study or sleep when he is up all night or out all night. It becomes so stressful for me, I move out. We still remain married, but we don't see each other that often. Unfortunately, after I move out…he parties more.

I am close to getting my degree in International Business from San Diego State University. It is finally my last year after ten years. Finishing school is the only thing that keeps me going, and of course, the dream that I will be healthy again someday.

I have a post-it on the wall above my desk that says:

| DON'T |
| GIVE |
| UP! |

I look at it often, and keep fighting. I live in an apartment close to the beach in Del Mar, California. It is so beautiful. I have surfed a little, but am usually not strong enough to paddle out. Most of the time, I don't even have enough energy to carry my surfboard down to the beach. From my apartment I have to walk down a steep trail to get to the beach. Just walking down to the beach totally exhausts me.

This is when the dolphins start cheering me up. When I first move there, I am so sad about moving away from Alex I say to God, "Okay God, if I see dolphins, then that is a sign that I'll be okay." And sure enough, I do! Another time, I am sitting on the beach crying so hard about Alex and my ill health. I look up and the dolphins are doing an amazing trick on top of the waves. It is so exciting... it is like being at Sea World. I can't believe it! I can barely see at first because my eyes are so filled with tears. About ten dolphins in pairs of two are skimming on top of the wave going parallel to the beach. Water is flowing up over their noses, along their backs and off their dorsal fins. It is so amazing! I really feel like they are putting on a show just for me.

This is an extremely hard year for me. A couple of times I am so tired and depressed, I feel suicidal. On the weekends, I go to the beach for a little while, then I go back to my bedroom and am exhausted. I just lie in bed. I am so lonely and frustrated that I don't have the energy or strength to go do anything fun. I don't have many friends either. It is almost impossible to have friends when I am too tired to do anything. I am always so tired.

There is a difference between being "Chronic Fatigue Syndrome" tired and a "healthy person" being tired. When normal healthy people are tired, they rest and then feel better, or they drink coffee or eat sugar, etc. Unfortunately, when you have CFS and you are tired, there is nothing that will give you energy. I can sleep all day long and still be tired! I wake up feeling like I haven't slept at all. I wonder if I actually do all those crazy things I dream about in my sleep - like run from monsters, ski down mountains, and run marathons! Because my polarity is reversed, I have static in my Central Nervous System which keeps me from entering into the deep levels of sleep that are necessary for rejuvenation. So I can sleep a long time and never feel rested!

Twice a week I take a night class, so I have a three hour break between classes. I am so tired, I get something to eat, then go to the parking lot and sleep in my car. I finally graduate from San Diego State University with a degree in International Business. Unfortunately, I am still too sick to get a job and use my degree. My mind is still foggy and some days are worse than others. My doctor from Mexico is amazed that I could actually attend school in my condition. I could handle going to classes 2 or 3 hours a day. My classes were in the afternoon, so I could sleep in. Some days if I was too sick to go to class, I would miss it. This was okay to do while I was in school, but it would not be okay to call in sick to work all the time. I also consumed large amounts of Ginkgo and Ginseng, which greatly helped my brain function in school, especially for a test or a midterm.

After being separated for a year, Alex convinces me to give him another chance. He promises he will stop using drugs. We rent a beautiful condominium on a cliff overlooking the ocean in Encinitas. I can watch the dolphins ride the waves and then jump out of them. Again they are there to cheer me up. Many times when we fight or I am upset, I go to the window or out on the balcony and the dolphins instantly change my mood and make me smile. What a blessing!

Unfortunately, Alex doesn't stop using drugs. I am so incredibly stressed out about the fact that he is still using drugs, and I am living with him. I am afraid he is going to die.

Because I am not physically, financially or emotionally capable of taking care of myself, I feel stuck in this situation. I start to feel suicidal again. I feel terrible for staying, but I don't have the strength emotionally or physically to leave. I am dying. I have given up the fight and sometimes I can actually feel my body poisoning itself.

Fortunately, I am seeing a doctor in Mexico who has been successfully treating patients with debilitating diseases. For $3,000 cash he sends my blood to Germany for an antigen treatment. I have an upper respiratory virus called Cytomegia Virus, the Herpes virus, and Staff bacteria in my blood besides the Epstein Barr virus. Fortunately, Alex has the money to pay for this special treatment from Germany, because it saves my life! At the lab in Germany, the doctor makes antigens for each virus I have. I then give myself shots daily for several months. This antigen triggers my immune system to fight off the viruses. After the first treatment from Germany, I ask my doctor if I am finished and he says, "Oh no - that batch just saved your life! You need another batch." The lab in Germany feels so sorry for me; they give me the next batch at a discount. This treatment is very successful. However, because my polarity is reversed my body is not able to permanently keep the viruses at bay. Also healing my emotional and mental body is necessary.

Up to this point I have tried everything! I have been on a strict diet for several years consisting of; no sugar, no wheat, no dairy, and no caffeine. I had all of my amalgam fillings removed. I do not wear any jewelry, make-up, or perfume. I do not eat or use any products that contain any chemicals. I am as "healthy and natural" as can be. However, a crucial factor in my move towards full recovery is my first session with an Energy Healer. I am fortunate enough to attend a lecture from Dr. Jaffe on Energy Healing and his School of Energy Mastery. I have an Energy Healing session with his wife. It is absolutely amazing. I had basically given up on God. I was down right mad at Him as well for "allowing" me to suffer for so many years!

During this session I close my eyes, while she guides me into my heart. My internal flame, my spirit is barely flickering. I feel so alone and so helpless. Then she asks me to imagine that God is in front of me and asks me to talk to Him. I don't actually hear Him or see Him. However, I definitely feel Him. I have a very deep knowing that He is there for me, and that He wants me to live. This connection I feel to God is so supportive. It completely restores my will to live and I no longer feel that I am totally alone and unsupported. I now have the strength, support, and courage to do what I need to do. She also points out that I need to eventually get away from Alex and the situation I am in.

Soon after, Alex goes on a two-day coke binge. I go to another town and stay in a hotel. I want to go to my mom's, but it is too far away and I am too weak to drive eight hours. Alex is so out of it that his friends are finally concerned about him. I tell him that I am leaving unless he gets help. My energy healer says she can try to help him if he goes to see her. So he does see her for a week, everyday, but he really needs a 30-day inpatient drug rehabilitation program.

Begin Healing my Mind and Spirit

A couple of months later, he goes to a halfway house. A part of me is relieved because I think his partying is over. I go to the basic training for the School of Energy Mastery. Dr. Jaffe has suggested that it will heal my CFS along with the treatments from Germany. The school consists of five two week sessions over two years. Alex is in a halfway house, so he can continue to work during the day. I attend the first session of the School of Energy Mastery. It is extremely helpful. I have learned by now that it is possible to heal myself and take care of myself and make it. Thank God!

This is when I first learn about self responsibility, which is taking responsibility for yourself, your feelings, and your actions, and not being a victim. This is crucial for me. The school also aids me in seeing more of my reality. I have been basically "going along for the ride" with Alex. I am not responsible for myself and I choose not to see everything. Therefore, I don't have to "deal" with everything. I learned this at an early age when I couldn't deal with my childhood situation. Back then I just went along for the ride because I had no choice. But as an adult I do! I can now see that Alex isn't getting his life together. He is partying again even though he constantly lies to me and swears that he isn't. It is really hard for me to accept. Somehow he is managing to keep using drugs and alcohol and to keep passing the drug tests at the halfway house.

I decide to move to Northern California, to start a business with my brother. Alex is going to be in the halfway house for a few more months. So we agree it will be good for me since we can't live together anyway. We are planning on seeing each other when we can, and he will then move to Northern California when his rehab is over.

The day before I am moving away, I'm packing up my stuff when the phone rings. I pick it up and a lady says, "Is this Margo Nagy?" "Yes" I reply. "This is Mrs.... from Scripts Hospital. Your husband has been in a bad car accident. Do you have a friend that can give you a ride here?" I hang up the phone thinking, wow, that was weird, why do I need a friend to drive me there...then I get sick to my stomach. I drive myself to the hospital and that lady takes me to her office sits me down, and says, "I'm sorry Margo, your husband Alex was in a really bad car accident... and died earlier this morning." Wow...what a shock! I am devastated! It turns out, he was taking Nitrous Oxide while driving at 9am in the morning. He was in the fast lane speeding as usual, when he must have passed out and veered off the freeway. His SUV rolled a few times, and he was thrown out of the sunroof that was open. He must not have been wearing a seat belt.

Thank God, I have started the energy healing school and am strong enough to handle this. After his death, I find out a lot of disappointing information about him. However, I still loved him deeply and it is a tragic loss. He had so much going for him, and he was only 33.

Although his death was a tragedy and a huge loss, it was also a blessing. My health begins to improve consistently after his death. I am no longer in such an intensely stressful situation with a very toxic and unhealthy person. I have also been unhealthy, however, I am continually growing and recovering. I am not looking forward to moving to Palo Alto in Northern California though. I am happy to be leaving Southern California, but I don't like living in or near cities! Unexpectedly…I receive some money from a life insurance policy. It is definitely a gift from God.

As I am driving to Northern California with all my stuff, I am pondering why I am going to live with my brother and start a business. That was my only alternative before Alex's death, but now I can go anywhere and do anything! It takes me a while to assess my own needs and desires. I have always been living my life for other people and wanting to make other people happy. I do what I think I "should" do or they think I "should" do. A part of me is wondering why I am going to start a business, which could be extremely stressful, and to live in a stressful environment. Of course, the part of me that wants to be successful and make lots of money.

However, deep in my heart I want to fully recover 100% and be healthy.

A month later after I have moved to Northern Ca., I'm laying face down, getting a massage, the first massage I have ever had, when I start really checking into my body and feeling what I need in order to get better. I see myself swimming in warm water and being in a warm, tranquil environment. I have never been to Hawaii, but my friend told me about it. I realize that my body needs to be pampered and nurtured. Kauai is just the place. At first it is really hard for me to let my brother down, but it is what I need to do. I want to get rid of CFS once and for all!

Major Improvement in my Health

So I move to Kauai in February of 1998. I find a nice little cottage on magical tropical land. It is so peaceful. The island is so beautiful and nurturing. There are so many places to go that take my breath away. Kauai's beauty sooths me. Some beaches I go to and cry about the loss of my husband and my struggle with CFS. Then I look around at paradise, the aqua blue water, the lush vibrant green foliage, the crisp blue sky, and am totally in awe of God's magnificent creation. I think "Wow, this is beautiful, 1 do want to live, life isn't that bad after all."

Fortunately, I don't have to work for a year, so I focus on healing myself and attending the School of Energy Mastery. Going to the school sessions is like eight hours of therapy a day. I deal with so many issues, negative behaviors, and aspects of myself. The two years of that school are incredibly transforming. Sometimes I feel like Humpty Dumpty that fell off the wall, shattered in millions of pieces, but I'm hanging in there and keep persevering through everything. I definitely have a lot of help and support from the healers/teachers from the school and my roommate and friend, Dr. Laura Smith.

Kauai is the perfect place for me to recover. The weather is always between 70-85 degrees year round on the North Shore. The island is only 56 miles around and not heavily populated. The major towns are small and traffic is minor in comparison to a major city. The pace of living is relaxed. The majority of the people who live there are relaxed as well. There is absolutely no smog! The ocean is not polluted. The overall environment is incredibly peaceful and beautiful. Although this island is small, it offers every type of climate and topography. Each side of the island is extremely different. The North Shore is lush and tropical. The East Shore is hot and desert like. Waimea Canyon is considered the mini Grand Canyon. At the top of the 3,000 ft. elevation, you feel like you are in Colorado. There are even pine trees!

While living on Kauai, I continue my Candida - free diet. Fortunately, I do not have to be as strict as I used to be.

My immune system is so much stronger I can handle occasional sweets and dairy. I try to exercise 30 minutes a day, at least three times a week. This consists of a walk on the beach, a swim in the ocean, a paddle on my surfboard, or a hike.

Almost Fully Recovered

In February of 1999 I finally receive a clean bill of health! I think I do anyway. I am so excited, I cry for joy and am filled with such gratitude for my recovery and the chance to fully live life again. This only lasts for a while, however because my polarity is still "reversed". Unfortunately…I continue to relapse again and again whenever I get too stressed.

My health has improved enough for me to work full time. About 1 year later I move to Mammoth Lakes, California to be closer to my family and friends, and to ski. My health is better than ever. I work full time for Mammoth Mountain Ski Resort. In the summer I hike and play tennis. After 2 years in Mammoth and two years living with my mom in Northern Ca. and working at Wyland Gallery in San Francisco, I miss Kauai so much, I move back.

While I'm back on Kauai I get my real estate license and begin selling real estate. In 2007 I get a fabulous job selling a new luxury condominium development in Poipu Kauai. It is a dream job. However, being "reversed" still affects me. I am always anxious, stressed and not able to do much after work. In the morning I am so anxious I can barely eat breakfast. I am just barely getting by. Some of the guys on my sales team ask me to go surfing after work but I am always too tired. After seven months, because the economy and the real estate market went to hell in a hand basket, they can only keep seven of the nine sales people on the sales team. They keep two who have been working for them before, and don't renew my contract.

Since I am finally making a lot of money, I decide to move back to Northern California where the job market is so much bigger to get another fabulous job. I know the real estate market is in the dumper... but I don't realize the entire economy is in such bad shape! After two months of searching for a fabulous job, I settle for a job as an assistant to a successful real estate agent in Tiburon, Ca. While she is in Paris at her Chateaux, I get to show her $65 million listing in Belvedere! She also has a $45M, and a few $5M - $16M listings. Again if the economy was not in such bad shape...I would be making a lot of money. However, as it turns out, nothing is selling and I can't cover the nut shell I have acquired. The stress of not having enough money has already taken a toll on my health. I am not functioning at 100% and start making mistakes at work that I would normally never make. I end up quitting because I am not making enough money.

After a couple more months of not getting a better job, I am really stressed. My friend has a diagnostic machine that reveals that I have the Epstein Barr Virus in my energy field. I am horrified! After all…I thought I was over that for good! At first I panic and think "Oh my God…here we go again. I'm going to be sick forever…I won't be able to work…I won't be able to take care of myself…what will I do?" I don't have anywhere to go and I am afraid I will be homeless! My mother lives in a retirement community so I can't live with her. Then I catch myself and remember that Epstein Barr is just a virus and that I know how to kill viruses with a zapper. Several years ago I had the fortune of being treated by Hulda Clark, an evolutionary scientist who invented a frequency generator called the zapper that kills viruses and bacteria. After realizing what I am actually doing, I take my power back from the whole "Chronic Fatigue Syndrome" mentality and label, and begin to use the tools I have for healing. However, because I haven't learned about "Chronic Reversed Polarity" yet, I still relapse.

If I'm not going to be making lots of money, I would much rather be in Kauai. So I call my ex-boyfriend and ask to stay with him while transitioning back to Kauai. He says sure…you can come live with me. At first this is a blessing, because I have relapsed so much, I am not able to work full time and need help getting back on my feet again. However, after 1 year of not working much, and not being able to live on my own and take care of myself financially, I find myself stuck again in an unhealthy living situation. Because my polarity is still reversed, I am not able to take the steps necessary to move out. I wake up in the middle of the night, completely paralyzed in fear just thinking about breaking up, moving out, and taking care of myself financially.

Full Recovery!

One day I am truly blessed while during a channeling session, my guides tell me about a master herbalist named Keith Smith. He discovered that the condition of "Chronic Reversed Polarity" is the cause of incurable diseases. He has been treating patients with all varieties of illnesses including terminal diseases for 30 years. He has also successfully treated many people with CFS. Finally, someone figured out why some illnesses and diseases are not curable! After taking his amazing herbal program for 6 months my polarity is un-reversed. Then I rebuild my adrenals and thyroid which have been so damaged over the years. Eventually, I am better enough to work more and am stable emotionally and mentally to move out and take care of myself financially. Because my central nervous system is more relaxed I am calmer and my body can handle more stress. So don't worry...if you are currently in an unhealthy relationship and or an unhealthy environment...when your polarity is normalized you too will have the strength both physically and mentally to take whatever steps are necessary to improve your life.

Now I wake up early. I actually feel rested when I wake up. I can go all day and do anything and feel strong and healthy. I am getting in awesome shape exercising everyday. I am skiing, surfing, hiking, doing yoga, and swimming in the ocean everyday! I'm much clearer, and able to express myself easily. Before, I had a hard time explaining myself. Since I am much calmer now, I don't get stressed out as easily and am more relaxed. Recently, I've noticed that my blood sugar is more stable. I can go longer without eating, and don't feel depleted, spaced out or ungrounded, like I used to feel if I didn't eat every 2-3 hours. Sometimes, I'm so happy I feel like I won the lottery! I am mostly grateful for my life and the amazing herbal program Keith Smith has developed. It is my mission to help others heal themselves so that they too can live there lives to its fullest!

I am living proof that you can heal from CFS! After 26 years of trying everything (many far out remedies and healing modalities I didn't even mention), I have finally discovered, thanks to Keith Smith, how to completely heal. **YES... YOU CAN HEAL FROM CFS AND DEPRESSION!**

* * *

II

CHRONIC REVERSED POLARITY

Chronic Reversed Polarity is the root cause of Chronic Fatigue Syndrome/CFS, Cancer, Depression, and other auto-immune diseases. The body is an electrical system. Electricity flows around the body creating an electromagnetic field. This electromagnetic field has a north and a south pole. Normally, your polarity spins clockwise. However, when this polarity is reversed, it weakens the immune system and causes static in the Central Nervous System resulting in illness and disease. Being chronically stuck in this reversed state keeps one from healing permanently. Thanks to Master Herbalist Keith Smith, his discovery 30 years ago reveals the key to healing "incurable" diseases such as CFS and depression.

What Causes It

Trauma and stress cause your polarity to become reversed. This can be physical, mental or emotional. When the body is overly stressed or traumatized, it's like jump starting a car and putting the cables on the opposing charges...you blow the circuits. The same is true with our bodies. Car accidents, divorces, deaths, bad relationships, stressful jobs, surgeries, flying, and other traumatic experiences are powerful enough to reverse one's polarity and change the direction your root chakra normally spins. I have had two surgeries, one on each shoulder. I have a screw in my left shoulder. Surgeries are definitely traumatic enough on your body to reverse your polarity. As you know, a magnet has a north and a south pole. If you stress a magnet enough…it will also reverse its poles. Some people's polarity naturally switches back to normal shortly after trauma, while others stay in this reversed state. There are exercises such as the cross crawl, and tapping on your Thymus which normalize your polarity. However, this only lasts 15 -30 minutes. Then your polarity switches back to being reversed.

What Happens

When your polarity is *chronically reversed* your body stops functioning normally. Your immune system is compromised and you contract whatever illness/disease you are genetically predisposed to such as Cancer, Chronic Fatigue Syndrome/CFS or other auto-immune diseases. Being in the chronic state of reversal, your body destroys itself and burns out. Because your body is not functioning normally, it is not able to hold any healing modalities such as chiropractic adjustments, homeopathy, acupuncture, or other alternative healing methods including conventional medical treatments. This is why people who have CFS get better temporarily, then relapse. In this reversed state there is a constant pull to stay reversed.

Being reversed causes static and chaos in your Central Nervous System, causing major sleep disorders. Deep levels of sleep such as Delta and Theta that are necessary for rejuvenation can not be reached. This lack of deep sleep leaves you fatigued and greatly impairs your memory, concentration and other normal brain function. Your brain also does not produce Serotonin which then causes depression. Lastly, this condition greatly inhibits the normal function of the immune system. So you can see that this Chronic Reversed Polarity condition wreaks havoc on your entire system.

How to Heal it

Fortunately this condition can be permanently normalized by taking Keith Smith's herbal program for 4-6 months. After your polarity is *un-reversed* you then rebuild your Adrenals, Thyroid and other parts of your body that were damaged. Our body is designed to heal itself. Once we get our polarity normalized and stable, it is then able to heal permanently and rebuild itself, even rebuilding brain synopses.

This herbal program consists of herbs that relax your Central Nervous System so your polarity can switch back to normal. Spirulina, a major part of this program has magnetic properties that hold your polarity in balance. The nice thing about this program is that you don't stop taking any medication you are currently taking. So if you are taking anti-depressants, you keep taking them until you feel better and don't need them anymore, of course under the guidance of the Doctor who prescribed them to you.

It is also necessary that your Atlas is in alignment. Because of many neck injuries, my Atlas would go out occasionally and I would have to have a chiropractor put it back in. It was challenging to find a chiropractor who could. The Atlas can be difficult to adjust properly. When it first came out, I was really dizzy for days. Now it is stronger and stable so it doesn't go out easily. If your Atlas is out for too long, it can cause your polarity to become reversed.

Results

After your polarity is un-reversed and you are able to sleep better and recharge your body and mind, you begin to think clearer. When you are clear, then you can work on healing your repressed emotions and old thought patterns (further discussed in Chapter III). With clarity you can now become aware of your thoughts, emotions, and beliefs. This allows you to catch yourself when an old limiting belief or program comes up, and release it. Remember…that was then and this is now. Now your polarity is normal, your body is functioning normally, and your mind is clear again. Now you can do whatever you want to do!

Since my polarity has been normalized, I see improvements in so many areas of my life! My depression is gone. There are moments of such immense joy unlike I have ever felt. Since my nervous system is relaxed, I am so much calmer and not anxious or nervous. I am more alive looking and people notice how healthy and vibrant I am. Thinking clearly allows me to express myself much easier. My concentration and memory improved tremendously. And of course my energy and stamina is amazing! I am skiing, surfing, hiking, doing yoga, and swimming in the ocean daily. I actually feel rested when I wake up in the morning, which I haven't felt in 28 years. Because of this, I even wake up earlier. After trying everything, and working so hard on myself, it is so nice to finally be functioning at 100% with all of my pistons firing. So hang in there…it is definitely worth the wait!

Additional Benefits

This amazingly powerful herbal program also raises your vibrational frequency. Everything vibrates at a certain frequency. The higher you vibrate…the better you feel. As you become more conscious, everything is clearer and more vibrant. Living on Kauai is already magical, but now the vibrant greens and blues are even brighter and I feel more connected to nature and the universe. I feel like I have been meditating in an ashram or sitting on top of a mountain for a year…and I only meditate 5-15 minutes a day. So not only are you feeling better physically… you are growing spiritually and naturally connecting more to God, the universe and your higher self.

✳ ✳ ✳

III

UNCONSCIOUS EMOTIONS, BELIEFS & PATTERNS

Identifying and releasing your unconscious emotions, beliefs, and patterns are essential for your complete recovery. Emotional or physical trauma that doesn't get processed gets stuck in your body and cells and manifests as either: pain, fatigue, depression, illness, or disease. Traditional Chinese Medicine believes that much of disease is caused by emotional repression. When emotions are not expressed, they are held in your organs and tissues inhibiting their normal, healthy function. These emotions form blocks which stop the natural flow of energy through your body, which can also reverse your polarity.

Energy tools such as Meridian Tapping (EFT), is an excellent way to uncover and release these repressed emotions and traumas. Hypnotherapy is also beneficial as it works with the subconscious. Some feelings are stuffed so deeply in our subconscious that we are not even aware they are there. Research shows that all subconscious patterns, beliefs, agreements and programming you take on in the first 7 years of your life, run 96% of your life! That is why positive thinking and affirmations don't work until you have released the limiting subconscious patterns and beliefs that are running your life.

Anger

When anger is unexpressed and unprocessed it can manifest as depression, compulsion, addiction, and can weaken your immune system. Research is now showing that 5 minutes of anger can weaken your immune system for 6 hours. While 5 minutes of loving feelings can stimulate your immune system for 6 hours.

Oh yes, the anger …I had a lot of anger stored deep in my subconscious: I was so incredibly angry with my father while growing up; consequently, I just chose to forget my entire childhood! As I mentioned earlier, my father was an alcoholic for most of my life. He was not happy with himself, and he projected his anger, shame, guilt and frustration on me. As a young child, I didn't know this, so I believed everything he said. For example, he would yell at me or tell me," You will never amount to anything! What is wrong with you?" He would yell at me for no reason and would imply that I was a bad person and that I was worthless, sometimes because I left the garage door open! I did not do anything to deserve this, and not everything he said was true. Unfortunately, at the time I believed him.

When I was young, I could not stand up for myself. Then when I was older, I was too afraid to stand up for myself. Consequently, I took on a lot of his anger and had generated a lot of my own. I also became extremely frustrated because I couldn't do anything about it.

Exercise:

When you have taken on someone else's anger or other emotion, you can close your eyes, imagine that person is right in front of you and give back their emotion that you took on. You can imagine you are handing it back in your hands, or imagine that it is energetically leaving your body and going back to theirs. Do whatever works best for you. You can also say out loud or to yourself, "I'm giving you back your anger, it is not mine and I don't want it. "Use your own words. This process is very empowering.

You can also do this with people you have given your power to. *Imagine you are standing in front of them, and say (to yourself), "I call my power back now.".* Unfortunately, most of the time we are not even aware that we gave our power away, or took on someone else's pain or emotion. For example; you can be in the check out stand at the grocery store and the clerk can be having a very bad day or be really upset. With out even talking to her, you can energetically take on her emotions. Next thing you know…you are walking out to your car and you feel upset! It's all about being aware of yourself and your emotions and being present.

I was so miserable living with my father. I felt that nothing I did was right and that nothing I did was good enough! I always wanted to prove him wrong. I actually looked into going away to a boarding school because it was so unbearable at times! It was also extremely overwhelming, and sometimes I felt so powerless and hopeless. I felt that I could not change anything.

Anger is a very powerful emotion. When it is not released, it is held in your body. Anger is usually held in the liver and causes the liver, or whatever organ it is affecting, to not function properly. During a lecture by Dr. Jaffe, he gave an example of a man who had been suffering from CFS for several years. Once he completely released all of his anger, his health dramatically improved!

Some of us do not like expressing anger, especially in front of anyone or directly to anyone. Sometimes we can be afraid of our own anger, and we are afraid we will lose control if we let it out. When I was in a school session at The School of Energy Mastery, a young man had so much anger to release that it took five men to hold him down. This is when it is helpful to be guided through it with a healer/practitioner.

How to Release Anger

With a healer/practitioner, or on your own, you can express anger through a silent scream. Sometimes I imagine that I am standing on a cliff in front of the ocean, and I'm screaming so loudly and powerfully that the water actually starts flowing back out into the ocean. It is as if my screams are intense winds! Or, you can scream into a pillow. My favorite release and the most beneficial for me, is to go out into nature alone and scream as loud as I can. This is really empowering. I never knew I could scream that loud and for that long! Kundalini Yoga is also an excellent way to release anger. If you have a DVD you can just do the exercises for releasing the anger and or only the ones you have enough energy for. My favorite is "Kundalini Yoga with Gurmukh" you can purchase it online at www.kundaliniyoga.org. Tapping is also an excellent way to release anger.

Now, after you have released all that anger, your body and your immune system can function better. Also, when someone or something makes you mad, you won't get triggered and have a volcano of anger ready to erupt! When you get triggered, that means a wound has been touched, or someone has touched a "soar spot". Research suggests that writing about our feelings and sharing them also strengthens our immune system.

Fear, Guilt & Shame

Unexpressed fear can result in anxiety disorders, insomnia, heart arrhythmias, sexual dysfunction and other stress related illnesses. Unexpressed guilt or shame may lead to self-neglect, compulsion, addiction, other self-destructive behavior and other chronic conditions. I had a lot of guilt and shame about being sick for so many years. Even after I recovered, this guilt and shame was still there in my subconscious affecting my self-esteem.

Forgiveness

It is really essential to forgive *yourself* for being sick. Forgive yourself for all of your mistakes, for anything you feel regret or shame about. Remember there is no right or wrong. We are here to make mistakes and learn lessons. It is all part of out experience here on earth.

It is also incredibly important to forgive others. Forgive everyone in your past that has ever hurt you or upset you. This will free up a lot of energy.

Exercise:

Say out loud the name of the person you want to forgive. Then say "I forgive you (dad) for hurting me intentionally and unintentionally. Please forgive me for hurting you intentionally and unintentionally."

This is great because you don't actually say it to them, but their higher self will get it. You can also write them a letter then read it out loud after calling on their higher self. Do this often whenever you feel a charge with everyone in your life; family members, friends, co-workers, bosses and boyfriends, etc.

Frustration

As you know…if you too are suffering from CFS, being sick for so long is incredibly frustrating especially after trying everything possible to recover. Not to mention the frustration of no one else understanding your predicament. I also had an enormous amount of frustration locked up in a box somewhere in my body! This frustration was from my childhood and my inability to do anything with my anger and other feelings. I grew up in a dysfunctional family where feelings were not expressed. It was as if there was an unspoken rule - and everyone pretended like everything was okay whether it was or not!

Unfortunately, my feelings of anger, sadness, disappointment, and shame were stuffed deep inside. If I ever did cry, it was alone in my bedroom, in my closet or outside in a hiding place. One time I had a nightmare and was so scared, I went to my mom and dad's room and sat in the corner crying. I was afraid to wake my father up for fear he would get mad at me. I have since learned that some of my fatigue is from keeping these feelings hidden and not dealing with them or expressing them. It actually takes a lot of energy to keep feelings locked up somewhere in our body. Now whenever I'm really tired for no obvious reason, I ask myself "what am I really feeling right now?" Sometimes I have been triggered by something and I am feeling an old emotion or memory. Or sometimes I'm sad and want to cry for no apparent reason. Again, something has touched an old wound that needs to be healed and released. When I think about all those 18 years of stuffing my feelings - that's a lot of feelings that need to be expressed.

My sister died of cancer at the age of 41. I believe that a major reason for this was her unexpressed emotions. They literally ate away at her. She was deaf and had a very challenging life. She was single and wanted a family so bad, but never met the right man. Despite all of her pain and frustration, she was always smiling as if everything was just fine. I didn't realize this until after her death.

Depression

Fortunately, un-reversing your polarity heals your depression. As I mentioned in Chapter II, when your polarity is reversed it causes static in your Central Nervous System which keeps you from going into the deep levels of sleep such as Delta and Theta. If you don't go into these levels of sleep, your brain does not produce Serotonin which then causes you to be depressed.

After several months of taking this herbal program after my polarity was un-reversed, I began sleeping better and eventually my depression lifted. It was amazing! I was still living in the same environment which actually was "depressing" to me before, but was no longer hopeless and overwhelming. It was just a situation I didn't want to be in any longer. I could see that I had a choice, and would be able to move out some day. I no longer felt the despair and hopelessness I had felt before.

One of Keith Smith's first cases treating clinical depression was a young boy who was 16. He was suicidal and had been in and out of mental hospitals. He was on lots of anti-depressants and other drugs for bi-polar disorder. He continued to take his medication while on the herbal program. When his polarity became un-reversed and he started to feel better he stopped taking the drugs and has been fine now for the past 11 years! If you are taking anti-depressants, don't stop. When you feel better, taper off until you don't need them anymore under the care of your doctor who prescribed them in the first place.

Feelings

Most people are not connected to their feelings. When you are not in touch with your feelings, then you don't "own" them. Owning your feelings means taking responsibility for your feelings and dealing with them rather than projecting them or dumping them on someone else. For example, when you get mad and don't own your feelings of anger, your anger then gets projected onto someone else, and they get mad.

This is common in relationships. Have you ever noticed that when your partner or friend comes home in a bad mood, next thing you know, you start arguing or you get in a bad mood? Next time you get in an argument, stop and ask yourself and the other person, "What is really going on here?

Whose anger or frustration is this? Where is it coming from? What is this really about?" Many times we start arguing for no real reason, then after the subject has changed... possibly a few times, you wonder, "How did this get started anyway?"

Sub-Personalities

We all have sub-personalities such as the critic, the pusher and the perfectionist. Each person has different sub-personalities. For me the perfectionist and the pusher pushed me so hard, I nearly went crazy! It is not easy being a perfectionist. I have a feeling most of you reading this right now...are perfectionists. During an energy healing session, the healer asked me to "retire" my perfectionist and critic. So...I am still working on that. Ha! I can now catch myself when I feel critical of myself and say, "Ok enough of you go back on vacation." Then remember everything is ok...I don't need to be perfect.

Beliefs

Whenever I would be really tired, or feel a little sick, I would almost automatically panic. I still have a hard time resting during the day or sleeping during the day. It always reminds me of being so sick and feeling paralyzed. Unfortunately, sometimes I still associate it with that. This is where the "re-programming" comes in, and "re-patterning". These beliefs that are formed in our subconscious need to be healed and released, so we can move on and let go of the past. After being sick for so many years, it was a major part of who

I was. I constantly found myself thinking "Oh no, I only had 5 hours of sleep, so I'll be tired or sick today", or "Oh I worked too long and hard, so now I'll be run down."

These are old beliefs that are no longer useful for me or true; therefore, they need to be released. The good news is…they can be re-programmed! Last winter I flew from Kauai to LAX at 9pm, then flew from LAX to Denver at 6am, drove to Vail, Co for 3 hours, skied for an hour, then went out to dinner! I hadn't slept much on the plane. However, I am so healthy now both physically and emotionally that my body was able to handle the lack of sleep. How exiting!

Our thoughts are so powerful. Our intentions are even more powerful! If you think you will be sick, then you will be. If you think you deserve to be unhappy, then you will be. So why not think and focus on what you want? This is explained more thoroughly in Chapter IX, The Power of Your Mind.

Tools to Release Emotions, Beliefs, and Patterns

Meridian Tapping (EFT)

Meridian Tapping also known as Emotional Freedom Techniques (EFT) is a form of psychological acupressure to stimulate traditional Chinese acupuncture points.

This is an excellent way to release these unconscious emotions, beliefs and patterns that are running your life. In fact by going through the tapping sequence you can discover your patterns and beliefs you have around an issue that you didn't even know. So when you start with a specific statement like, "Even though I'm afraid to be successful, I love and accept myself." When you go into those feelings – more feelings and beliefs may come up around this. For example, you may remember why you are afraid to be successful.

This tool is really powerful and can be used on so many things….pretty much everything! You can use it daily. Every time a negative emotion comes up like anger or sadness. Stop and start tapping! If you are having a hard time doing it by yourself. There are experts in this field of (EFT) who can help you. Check the Resources section. Especially in the beginning it is very helpful to have an expert or an outsider to walk you through it and give you the correct language to get to the cause and release it successfully. It gets easier the more you do it and play around with it. I also recommend the website www.thetappingsolution.com. Each issue may take more rounds than others.

On page 53 is a **diagram** of the **tapping points**.

Here are some issues I tapped on:

- My pattern of doing things and jobs when I really didn't want to do them and then felt resentful and frustrated.
- My co-dependent pattern of taking care of everyone else's needs before mine and feeling responsible for others.
- Released all my anger and frustration about being sick for so many years.
- Released all of my shame and guilt about borrowing money from my family and not being able to pay them back yet.
- Released "my story" of pushing myself and doing so much that I was always tired, overwhelmed, stressed, frustrated and not having fun or following my passion and creating my dreams
- Released all of my cultural agreements such as the need to be busy and overwhelmed, or that I must struggle and work hard to make money.
- Released all of the trauma from my cellular memory from; car accident, ski accidents, Alex's death, surgeries, and other emotional traumas.

Tapping Points

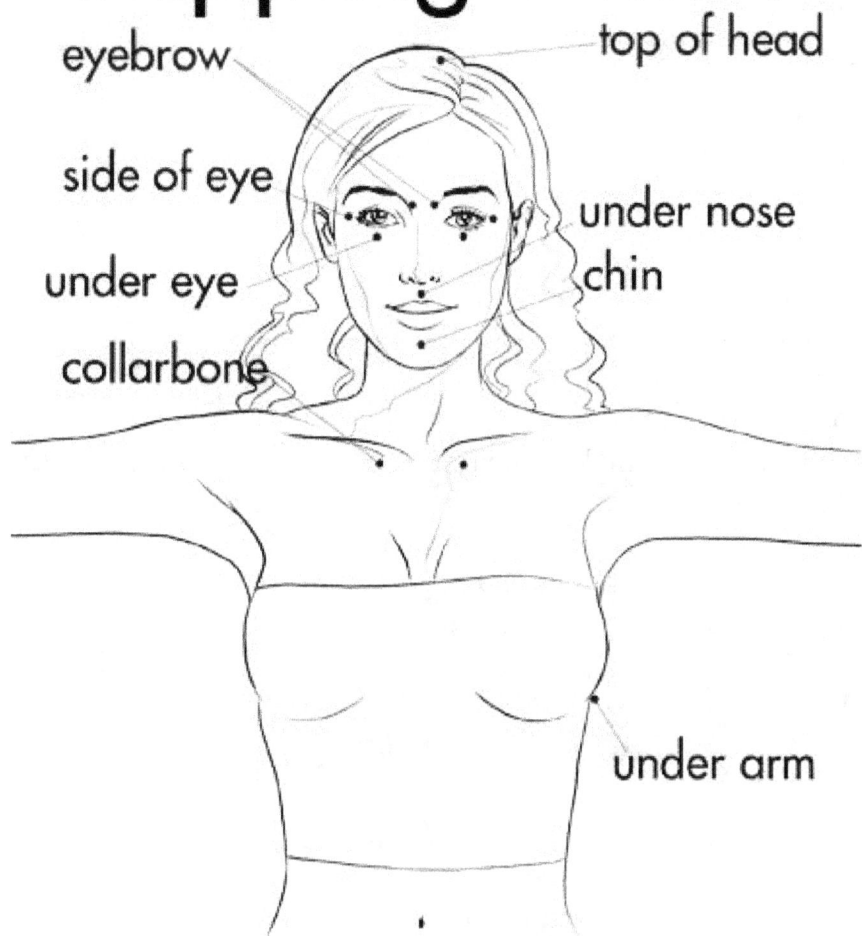

eyebrow

top of head

side of eye

under nose

chin

under eye

collarbone

under arm

www.TheTappingSolution.com

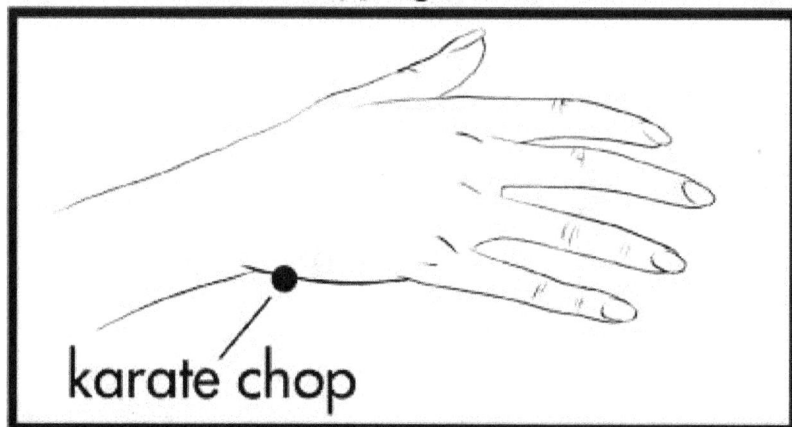

karate chop

You can tap on either side of your face, with either hand and can go back and forth.

Here is a sample script:

First ask yourself, "How do I feel about this statement on a scale from 1 – 10?"

Round 1

Karate chop – Even though I have this pattern of doing what I don't want to do, I love and appreciate myself.

Karate chop – Even though this pattern of doing what I don't want to do make's me resentful and frustrated, I love and appreciate myself.

Karate chop – Even though I have this pattern of doing what I don't want to do, I love and appreciate myself.

Eyebrow – I always do what I don't want to do.

Side of eye – I feel resentful and frustrated.

Under eye – Why do I do things I don't want to do?

Under nose – I'm afraid I'll get in trouble if I don't.

Under chin – I'm afraid someone will get upset if I don't do what they want.

Under arm – I hate feeling this way.

Collar bone – I hate doing what I don't want to do.

Top of head – I am tired of doing what I don't want to do.

*Take a deep breath.

Test how you feel now on a scale from 1 – 10.

Round 2

Karate – Even though I still have this pattern of doing what I don't want to do, I realize that I don't have to anymore.

Karate – Even though I have this pattern of doing what I don't want to do, I see it no longer serves me.

Karate - Even though I have this pattern of doing what I don't want to do, I am ready to release it.

Eyebrow – I see that it is not true.

Side of eye – I see that this pattern no longer serves me.

Under eye – I am now ready to release this pattern.

Under nose – I now release this pattern of doing what I don't want to do.

Under chin – I release all of my resentment and frustration.

Collar bone – I now choose to do only what I want to do.

Under arm – It is safe for me to do only what I want to do.

Top of head – I am now only doing what I want to do and it feels good.

* Check to see how you feel.

You may need to do another round or two.

Running Programs

We also run programs that are not healthy or positive. For example; one of my programs is "poor me". I get into this poor me, victim mode and I feel like I can't have what I want or do what I want. If I allow myself to stay in it…it is paralyzing! Fortunately, I am aware of it now and can catch myself. About a year ago, I woke up and was upset about losing my job, when I got this vision of me starting the day by picking up these huge heavy rocks to carry around with me all day. One rock said, "poor me" and it was so big and heavy! Then I imagined what it would be like carrying all this weight and negative draining energy around with me all day and realized why I didn't want to get out of bed. Now I imagine how nice it would be to drop those heavy rocks and let go of all the anger, frustration and resentment…and be over with it! Wow…what a weight lifted.

Our emotions can be so draining, and don't serve any purpose to hold on to them like this. Yes, you should feel your initial feelings…then let them go (or tap on them)…and move on. Each moment and each day is an opportunity to create whatever you want.

Conclusion

Now you can see how powerful these unconscious emotions, patterns and beliefs are. We don't even have to be consciously aware of them… for them to greatly affect our body, mind and spirit. This is why it is so important to heal the emotional body as well as the physical body! You can do this by tapping daily and if necessary, work with a hypnotherapist or EFT practitioner that can access your subconscious so you can see what beliefs and programs are really running your life. When you have released all of your limiting emotions, beliefs, and patterns… you are then free to create radiant health and happiness.

* * *

IV

STRESS

Stress is what causes you to get sick when your polarity is reversed. When you experience intense or constant stress you succumb to whatever illness, condition or disease that you are predisposed to. The amount of stress you feel in any situation is from your reaction to it. Many times this is unconscious and may be a "knee jerk" reaction. Fortunately we do have control over how we react to stress and deal with it. We can eliminate some stresses, learn to react differently to stress, and by meditating, meridian tapping and exercising regularly we can handle stress much easier. In this chapter, I give you some examples of stress along with tools to manage your stress and reprogram the way your body reacts to stress.

Environmental Stress

Environmental stress comes from our environmental surroundings. Cities are filled with this kind of stress. For example, traffic, loud noises, people everywhere and concrete everywhere. There is an over all "busy and fast paced" energy in a city. Many people like this kind of fast paced energy and actually thrive on it. While others who are sensitive or sick are stressed and negatively affected. When I was sick I couldn't handle being in a city. I would get nervous, anxious and tired.

At one point, I couldn't even go out to dinner in a busy and loud restaurant, because it was too stressful. Now that I am healthy - it doesn't bother me - I don't even notice it anymore.

Another form of environmental stress is smog, which is harmful to your body especially when you are sick. In cities there is an average of 10% oxygen in the air. In suburbs there is 20% oxygen. In some cities like Mexico City, the smog is so bad, there is a high percentage of people who have chronic bronchitis. Some people even ware masks to keep the smog out of their lungs.

Cold weather is another form of environmental stress. Our bodies have to work much harder to keep warm in cold weather. When you are healthy, this is not a problem, but when you are sick, all of your energy is going towards healing your body and aiding in all of its systems functioning properly. When I was sick, my doctor told me not to go to the mountains in the winter. Even when I received a clean bill of health, he told me not to live in the cold for 6 months.

Emotional Stress

Emotional stress can come from working in an environment that is hostile and or stressful. Working under pressure constantly can be hard on your body and your emotional state. Emotional stress is high if you are in a relationship that has a lot of conflict, blame frustration, guilt, or abuse. Being in a relationship with an addict or alcoholic is extremely stressful. This is probably the most stressful and harmful situation, because the emotional abuse and emotional stress is so unhealthy. Beginning the day after my addict husband died - my health improved daily, because so much emotional stress was eliminated from my life. We can also be stressed from our emotions. Experiencing loss, change or disappointment can be very emotional. Financial stress was major for me, but now that I am healthy and have cleared my limiting beliefs and patterns, I am attracting more money into my life easier.

Physical Stress

Physical stress can come from physically pushing yourself too hard. Like working long hours and not giving your body enough rest, or working out, playing tennis or skiing too long when you are tired. I know that when I am skiing, if I keep skiing after I am tired, I am much more likely to have an accident and hurt myself. One time I was skiing in Utah. It was my last run. I was overly exhausted and should have quit an hour earlier. I was just going on a beginner road when my ski tips crossed. I lost my balance and was too tired to catch myself. I fell on my head and sprained my neck. Now when I'm tired...I stop skiing.

Mental Stress

Mental stress is something we can actually create ourselves. This stress comes from what is going on in our mind - what we are thinking. Is your mind busy? Is it constantly thinking and racing? This is stressful on the body. Our mind can push us and criticize us all day long - (You should do this. You should do that. What are you doing? That is not right! You are stupid. You need to try harder!) Does this sound familiar? This constant bombardment of negative self-talk can physically ware your body down. Until we become aware of this self- talk, we may not even realize it exists. I didn't realize how bad mine was until I consciously became aware of it. It is so much better that now I can catch myself and choose to think more positive, supporting and loving thoughts. You can also accomplish this. Meditation is a great way to be aware of your thoughts, and to give your mind a rest.

Expectations

If you are like me...you have many expectations of yourself. You may also feel that you have many expectations from other people. If you do...let them go right now! We are responsible for ourselves only. Deep down, only we know what is best for us. You may not be in touch with this part of yourself yet, and that's ok. In this book I give you tools and exercises to hear your own guidance and follow your intuition. So that after you normalize your polarity and strengthen your connection to your higher self and your inner guidance, then you will know what is best for you. This is also related to being co-dependant, which is feeling responsible for others and putting other's needs in front of yours.

Back to the expectations of yourself, yes we come into this world with lots of expectations and illusions about what we think we are "supposed" to do. This is based on the cultural programming we pick up about comparing ourselves with The Jones's, our neighbors, or people on TV and in magazines. The good news is that we are NOT supposed to be like them or anyone. We came here to this planet with our own individuality and our own unique way to communicate with others and spread our love and light. And there is no right or wrong way to do this. So for now...please lose all of your expectations (except for the one of you healing and being healthy and happy of course). All the other ones are not important anymore. When you get better some may still be, but for now, let's take all the pressure off so you can just relax and heal. You also may be a totally different person when you heal so you may have different expectations and definitely healthier ones. Know that when your polarity is normalized. You will think clearly. When you are healthy and feel better your life will be better in so many ways.

A major misconception and illusion that most of us have is that we are supposed to accomplish certain things like; be a good mother or father, wife, husband, employee, etc. And really...we came here to figure out how to be healthy and happy so that we can smile at a stranger and spread our love and light. When we are peaceful and vibrating high, we are a positive influence on others.

So let all of your expectations go, and love yourself right now, even being sick. You still have love and light in you – nothing and no one can ever take that away from you! Keep loving yourself as much as possible and see love in others and in everything.

Also…when you do get better, there is nothing expected of you. There is no loss of time that needs to be made up. There is nothing to prove to anyone. Just be happy. Follow your heart. Connect to God, your higher self and love, and emanate your love and light out into the world. That is what the planet needs right now and it is so easy. It is as easy as smiling at a stranger, meditating and connecting to that love inside you and imagining it pouring out of your body and out into the world.

Tools to Manage Stress

Fortunately, one of the herbal formulas in the herbal program to un-reverse your polarity, relaxes your Nervous System, so you feel much more calm and peaceful. However, these tools will also support your body in managing stress and staying in balance.

Meridian Tapping

Meridian Tapping/(EFT) is an excellent way to release stress either while it is occurring or is already stored up in your body. As I mentioned in Chapter III, this is a technique that you can do on your own anytime, anywhere. Tapping can actually reprogram the way your body reacts to stress!

Here is a sample script for releasing stress when it is occurring and stopping your body's "flight or fight response".

Round 1

Karate chop point - Even though I am stressed right now, I love and accept myself

Karate chop point - Even though I feel stress right now, I love and accept myself

Karate chop point - Even though I am totally stressed right now, I am ok.

Eyebrow - I'm really stressed

Side of eye - This stress

Under eye - I feel overwhelmed

Under nose - I don't know what to do

Under chin - I hate feeling so stressed

Collar bone - No matter what happens, I will still be ok

Under arm - I can release this stress if I want

Top of head - Maybe everything will be fine

Round 2

Karate chop point - Even though I am still stressed, I love and accept myself

Karate chop point - Even though I feel stress, I can choose peace

Karate chop point - Even though I feel stressed, I am ready to release it

Eyebrow - I am now ready to release this stress

Side of eye - I release this stress

Under eye -I am releasing this stress from my body now

Under nose - I am fine whatever happens

Under chin - I choose peace

Collar bone - I am relaxed now

Under arm - It feels good to relax

Top of head - I trust that everything is ok

Sometimes it may take more than 1 or 2 rounds depending on the complexity and severity of an issue. And the great thing is that other issues come up during this. So you can continue to tap on those. For example, as you start tapping on your stress then you realize you also have fear and then you see you have a pattern of attracting this kind of stress so you keep tapping on all this related issues! You can use your own words and say whatever is coming up for you. Also…after you have been doing this for a while, you can just tap on 1 or 2 points and that will stop your body's stress response. For example, a man was getting on an airplane and he felt some anxiety coming on, so as he was putting his carry on in the compartment above his seat, he started tapping on his collar bone. This triggered his body to start relaxing. You could then sit down and tap some more and just say "I'm ok, everything is ok, I'm safe, there is nothing to worry about, etc."

Meditation

Meditation is a very affective way to manage stress. Meditation is a process of relaxing your body and mind to achieve immense peace and to connect to your higher self (your inner wisdom) and to God. When you have attained a quiet state and you are connected to your inner wisdom - you can receive messages. It is in this state that your entire body rests, heals, and repairs itself at a very deep level. During meditation your body actually stops aging It has been scientifically proven that regular meditation can add 5-20 years to your life. I have been meditating for 10 years now and everyone I meet thinks I am 10 years younger than I am!

How to Meditate

To meditate, sit in a chair with your back straight and your feet on the ground shoulder width apart. Place your hands on your thighs with your thumb touching your first finger, or your hands on your lap, one in front of the other. You can also sit on the floor on a pillow with your legs crossed. Keep your back straight. Close your eyes and begin to breathe deeply and slowly. Put all of your awareness and focus on your breathing. Feel the air moving up from your stomach to your lungs and feel your chest expanding. Breathe in through your nose and out through your mouth. Listen to the air gently flowing through your nose and out your mouth. Allow your shoulders to relax, then the rest of your body part by part. If you notice tension somewhere then breathe into the area and allow it to melt and deeply relax. If your mind is busy and you have many thoughts entering your mind-just let them move on and don't hold on to them. Bring your awareness back to your breathing.

Mantra repetition is very helpful to clear your mind. This is done simply by repeating a mantra over and over. After awhile your mind quiets down. It may take 20-30 minutes when you are staring. Or you can focus on your breath.

You can also create a space in your house for meditation. Lighting a candle and burning incense can create a relaxing atmosphere. When you meditate in the same place regularly this space holds the energy of peace and relaxation that your meditating creates. This also aids in your meditating process. Meditating in nature is very conducive, and meditating during a full moon is incredibly powerful.

Now I listen to the new CD from Abraham-Hicks called "Getting into the Vortex." I find that when my mind is especially busy - listening to this CD is so much easier than trying to quiet my mind on my own. After a while your body will become "trained" to meditate. Eventually, you will be able to be anywhere and close your eyes and immediately tap into the peace and relaxation of meditation. That is what was so amazing about swimming with the dolphins in the wild. As soon as my head was under the water and the dolphins were swimming around me – I felt like I was in a meditative state.

Meditation is also helpful to relieve anxiety. When you feel anxious or nervous, you can close your eyes for a couple of minutes and take some deep breaths. This will calm your body down physically and mentally. After meditating enough to attain that extremely peaceful and relaxing state, whenever you want you can connect to this wonderful feeling. I was skiing one day and riding on a chairlift that was going up to the top of a very steep expert run. I was tired and started to feel anxious, so I closed my eyes and focused on my breathing and my mantra. After only 2-3 minutes - I opened my eyes and felt relaxed and peaceful. Meditation is also an excellent way to connect to God and your higher self, which I speak about more in Chapter VIII, "Connecting to God and Your Higher Self".

Long Term Benefits of Meditating

The more time you spend meditating and being in the love and the ultimate truth, the easier it becomes to connect to, and the easier it becomes to stay connected to throughout the day. Meditating regularly also builds up a reservoir of peace. When you have been meditating daily, your resistance to stress is much higher. If you are in a stressful situation it doesn't affect you as much if you have been meditating. A few years ago, I had a very stressful job. I was actually doing the job of two people. I noticed that if I didn't meditate for 4 or 5 days, I would snap so easily. Everything would stress me out much more! Some stressful situations - I couldn't even deal with. However, when I was meditating daily sometimes morning and night, I could handle anything. It became so obvious. For one month I was having such a hard time even going to work. I felt like I was on the verge of a nervous breakdown. The only way I could go to work was to listen to my meditation CD for at least 20 minutes before I went to work. Then on the way to work, in my car, I would chant to one of my chanting CDs. It became very clear to me how important and beneficial meditating had become for me. Now I notice if I have gone just one day without meditating. As I mentioned earlier, even meditating for only 5-10 minutes is so helpful!

Chanting

Chanting has great healing power. Chanting gets you in touch with the love within you and all around you. Pure ecstasy and bliss can be reached when chanting. Sometimes my entire body tingles with ecstasy. After chanting you are in a very deep meditative state, which allows you to continue meditating effortlessly. Chanting can also change your mood. One day I was depressed and didn't want to do anything, but I also didn't want to feel so depressed! So I chanted for 40 minutes. When I was finished - I felt happy. This wonderful feeling stayed with me throughout the rest of the day and night. Even at work that night I felt extra chipper.

Like meditation - when chanting it may take 20-30 minutes to get to a peaceful and happy state. I remember when I first started chanting with a group of people in Kauai. In the beginning I had a hard time. The very first time - I kept thinking, "why am I saying all of these words in another language over and over? What am I doing here? This is a waste of my time." Then in the last 5-10 minutes I started smiling and feeling immense peace and bliss! One time I was so ecstatic - I started laughing. Chants usually start out very slow, then they speed up. This chant had sped up so much that it was tongue twisting trying to sing the words so fast. I found this to be so funny - I couldn't stop laughing.

The nice thing about chanting is that it always seems to "win" in the battle of our bombarding thoughts. It may take awhile and you may be tempted to stop or go to sleep, but every time - at some point your busy mind surrenders and you reach an incredible state. The background music of some chants make me want to dance. One time I was chanting with headphones on that were plugged into my stereo. The chant had sped up and the beat was fast. I was standing up and bouncing my head back and forth from one side to the other. I began to whip my head back and forth with so much momentum – my headphones flew off of my head! I laughed hysterically. To order chants on CD or tape you can call the Siddha Yoga Center at (888)422-3334 or online at www.bookstore.siddhayoga.org.

Yoga

Yoga is a gentle exercise of movement. By slowly moving from one pose to another, you stretch and strengthen your muscles. Holding the different poses requires concentration, balance and strength, which greatly improve with practice. Yoga also gets you in touch with your body, and can produce a meditative state. Yoga ultimately balances your body, mind and spirit.

Physically yoga is extremely beneficial. According to the American Yoga Association Beginners Manual, the yoga exercises provide maximum flexibility and strength to the skeletal, muscular and nervous systems. Some poses massage internal organs and improve circulation. Over time the nervous system is strengthened which results in increased concentration and a more stable emotional nature. The stretching of muscles improves blood flow, which provides more oxygen to all parts of the body. The focus on breathing during yoga helps release stress and increase energy.

Some yoga poses are strenuous, and some yoga classes and videos can be challenging. However, there are classes and videos that are more gentle. Some mornings I do the first 10-20 minutes of a video called, "Yoga Practice for Energy with

Rodney Yee." The first 10 minutes are nice and easy stretches laying on the floor. Yoga classes are usually one - one and a half hours long, which may be too much. However, with your own yoga video you can do as little or as much as you want. I have found that even as little as 10 minutes a day has greatly benefited me. I have better balance when I ski. I have noticed that my body is much more flexible and it actually heals from physical strain or soreness much quicker. It has become a very important part of my day. I play the video first thing every morning. It relaxes me and puts me in a good mood to start the day. It is also improving my posture. My entire life I have been slouching. I didn't realize how badly I was - until I saw myself in a mirror and was horrified! Now after doing yoga, which is strengthening my spine, standing up straight is much easier and sometimes effortless.

If you have never done yoga before, I recommend going to a beginner yoga class or having a personal yoga instructor come to your house to make sure that you are doing the poses correctly. You don't want to be doing them wrong or injure yourself. Then you can buy a beginner's yoga video and a yoga book with pictures of the poses. And remember to only do as much as your body can handle. With a book you can pick out 1 - 4 poses and do them each day. Or with a video like the one I use that is broken down into 10 minute segments, just do one segment or two.

Deep Breathing

As I mentioned earlier, breathing is a very important part of yoga. When breathing deeply, oxygen is increased to the brain in several ways. Studies have shown that yoga actually increases vital capacity of the lungs over a period of several months.' Breathing exercises are great especially when you are too tired or ill to do other exercises. By deep breathing you are still increasing the oxygen flow throughout your body as you do when exercising.

Breathing Exercises

When breathing properly, correct posture is necessary. It is important to keep your back straight. While breathing in allow your belly to relax and expand with air. Continue to bring that air up and into your chest feeling your chest expand. Then gently exhale as slowly as you inhaled. After some practice you can try to inhale for 10 seconds and exhale for 10 seconds. Don't hold your breath. Keep the breathing smooth and balanced. In the beginning you may become lightheaded. Stop, and try again. Eventually the lightheadedness will go away. You may want to use earplugs, which allow you to hear your breath more and concentrate better.

Pranayama Breathing: *Sit comfortably in a chair, with your back straight. Take your right thumb and place it over your right nostril. Breathe through your left nostril and exhale through your right nostril closing your left nostril with your right first finger. Do*

73

this for 10 20 minutes. This oxygenates your brain resulting in alertness and focus.

*These are just a couple of exercises. Many more can be found in yoga books and meditation books.

Exercise

Exercise is another excellent way to manage stress. Sometimes a meditative state can be reached while jogging or walking. Exercise can also be fun. It feels good to be outside in the fresh air and the sun. It has been proven that we actually need a little bit of sun to produce vitamin K. For me, a little bit of sun cheers me up and feels so good.

Exercising is also a great way to either take your mind off things or to think about your life. Sometimes when I'm walking I easily and effortlessly work out problems or come up with solutions. Many times I'm creatively inspired and come up with new ideas or revelations. I see my life and "the bigger picture" more clearly. It can also be a great way to release emotions.

My oldest sister is so healthy and in great shape - despite all of the stress she encounters! She is 62 years old, and she has been running on the beach and working out in the gym consistently since her early twenties. Exercise produces endorphins that elevate your mood. I noticed that when I ran - even for only 5 - 10 minutes, I felt incredibly better! All of a sudden, everything seemed fine, not so hopeless. I felt happy and my whole outlook on life improved! If you can't run, try breathing really deep for 10 - 20 minutes as if you were running. This may give you the same affect, or jumping on a mini trampoline

If you are too tired or weak to vigorously exercise go for a walk. Even a 5 or 10 minute walk will benefit you. For a few months I was so weak - I couldn't go for a walk. As soon as I had a little bit of strength, I started walking, sometimes for only 10 minutes. Or do some yoga stretches. The stretches on the floor are great because you are lying on the floor, which requires less energy. Dancing is another way to get the blood and oxygen flowing. Put on your favorite music and dance! Go ahead don't be shy - nobody is watching. Most importantly have fun and remember that even a little can go a long way.

Being in Nature

Being in nature is another great way to relieve stress and to heal your self. Nature can be so soothing and nurturing. That is why the north shore of Kauai was so healing for me. When I am there, the magical surroundings engulf me. The land, the air, and the water are filled with healing power. As I stand on a sandy beach gazing into the turquoise blue water - peace and tranquility fill every cell of my body. The warm crystal clear water invites me to feel its soothing touch. As I enter the soft water, I feel supported and free. I am purified and healed. As I look around I see bright green everywhere. Everything is so lush and colorful. I feel as though I am being cuddled by these vibrant green surroundings.

Being in nature is also so quiet. You are able to relax and spend time with your self. When I was living in Mammoth Lakes, a ski resort in California, in the summer I would go on a hike everyday. Some days when I would be feeling sad and lonely, I would go for a hike. As soon as I started hiking - I would feel better. Next thing I knew, I would be skipping through the forest with a big smile on my face. The trees are so nurturing to me. I don't feel alone when I am in the mountains. I feel so connected to nature and to God. One day, I hiked to a lake that was so magical. Aspen trees shades of yellow, green and orange shimmering in the sunlight surrounded the deep blue water. "This is what I live for," I thought.

When I am in nature, I am also so inspired. It allows me to contemplate my life from a different, new and expanded perspective. I can reflect on my life and where I am going. There are no distractions, and my stress just melts away.

Conclusion

As you can see, stress is an inevitable part of our lives. Not only is it important to learn how to handle stress, it is equally important to control and manage the way you create stress. Everyone reacts to each situation differently with various levels of stress or no stress. Meditating, Meridian Tapping and exercising regularly keep you in a more relaxed state so that your body physiologically reacts less to stress. However, the key is to learn how to let go of attachments, expectations, go with the flow, and completely trust that everything is happening in divine order. Fortunately, after your polarity is normalized and your body rests and rejuvenates itself…your body and mind naturally can handle stress much better!

' Funderburk, R.K. Science Studies Yoga. Glenview, 111. Himalayan Publications, 1977

* * *

V

ENERGY HEALING

Energy healing was an important part of my full recovery. What is energy? Everything is energy. Our body is a field of energy. Emotions, memories, beliefs and thoughts are all energies, which can be held in the body forming blockages and causing imbalance. With Energy Healing, we can reveal these blockages and heal them. When energy flows properly throughout the body, all internal parts of the body function perfectly, resulting in radiant health.

Different Types of Energy Healing

Different types of Energy Healing have been around for thousands of years. Acupuncture, Acupressure and Reiki release blocks of energy in the body and balance the natural flow of energy. Chinese Chi Gong is a technique used to heal, maintain wellness, and prevent illness by balancing the body's energy flow. Some other forms of Energy Healing include: Therapeutic Touch, Jin Shin Jyutsu, Hypnotherapy and Healing Touch.

Energy Healing is not magic. Hands on Healing and Reiki have a similar affect as Acupuncture. The human energy field is a bio electromagnetic field. During a healing session the healer's bio magnetic field interacts with the client's bio magnetic field causing changes to occur in the client's electric field. When energy blocks are released, the client's chemical balance is changed at the cellular level and chemicals are released, resulting in physiological changes. The cell's structure and function actually change.

Voice Dialogue

Voice Dialogue is a technique used, which was developed by Hal Stone, PH.D. and Sidra Stone, PH.D. Voice dialogue involves verbal communication between the healer and the different voices/sub-personalities of the client. Some common voices are: the Critic, the Pusher, the Protector, and the Saboteur. Each client has his/her own set of voices/sub-personalities. Often these voices have been taken on from someone else, like a parent.

During voice dialogue we can see from where these voices are coming. Then we can see what each voice needs and what its purpose is. Some of these voices can be healed. Some voices will always be a part of us; however, when we know from where they originate, and we know that they are not of the truth, then we can choose to filter out their influence. For me, one of my most influential voices was the Pusher. This voice constantly pushed me so hard that I over did everything and stressed my body too much, leading to illness. During an energy healing session I was able to find out that this voice was from my Dad, and it was seeking to be loved. So whenever I noticed that I was pushing myself, I would stop and think, "Oh, this is really about my dad, and I don't have to keep pushing myself in order to be loved."

Hands on Healing

Magnetic and Radiatory Healing are done through the hands. The healer places his/her hands over the area of the body that needs to be healed. The hands are placed approximately 6 inches off the body, which is called the etheric body. Using Magnetic Healing the energy is pulled magnetically from the client's body. This energy is taken out of the client's energy field and dissolved into the light, which is like a column of light coming down from above. Sometimes energy is radiated out from the healer's hands and into the client's body. This is called Radiatory Healing. These forms of healing assist the energy to move out of the client's body. Sometimes these methods are used to bring the client's awareness into an energy when the client is having difficulty connecting to the energy.

For example, when I was doing an energy healing session on a client who had recently had a mastectomy, my hand was guided to her chest. I was radiating energy to stimulate the blocked energy (anger) in this area. My hand could feel the heat rising from this area. I then felt her pain and anger. By keeping my hand a couple of inches above this area, the client could then bring her awareness here and get in touch with the pain and anger that she had previously repressed.

Reiki

Reiki is a Japanese healing technique which is also used for stress reduction and relaxation. The Reiki practitioner guides the universal life force energy throughout the client's body. This life force energy also goes to wherever there are blockages in the body and releases them so the client's energy is able to flow smoothly. Pain can be eliminated and profound healing can occur with this powerful technique. The practitioner's hands are either placed directly on the body, up to several inches off the body, or can be done over long distance.

If you become a Reiki practitioner you can do it on yourself. I am Reiki certified and do it on myself often. It works fast when I have an upset stomach. I place my hands on my stomach, and within minutes I start feeling the energy moving and in 5-10 minutes, my stomach ache goes away! Animals also respond miraculously, probably because they don't have any limiting beliefs about the power of such energy healing techniques. I did Reiki on a 14 year old dog that could not jump into my car, and was limping badly. After just a few 20 minute Reiki sessions…he was jumping in and out of the car on his own and running up and down the hiking trails!

During an Energy Healing Session

During an energy healing session you are guided into
your body and your subconscious to reveal issues, beliefs,
emotions, and illusions that are holding you back and/or
creating illness. In the beginning you close your eyes, relax,
and breathe deeply. By breathing deeply into your belly, you
become in touch with your body and grounded. You also
become aligned with your true self/higher self and with God.
You are then guided into your feelings so you can really
experience them. Some feelings are stuffed so deep inside, that
we are not consciously aware that they even exist.
Unfortunately, wherever they are being held in the body, they
are harming that area and blocking the natural flow of energy.
Although, when you bring your awareness to this hidden
energy, you can fully experience it and understand why it is
there. When you feel that you no longer have a need for it and
you have learned your lesson regarding this energy, then you
can release it. When it is released, healing occurs at a cellular
level, affecting the DNA. This is why energy healing is so
powerful and transforming. After an energy is released, the
area is filled with white light and love. When a negative belief
is released, it can be replaced with a new empowering belief
and/or the truth.

Awareness is brought to the desired energy sometimes
revealing it in the subconscious. The client can then see why
the energy is there, what the need is, and what is needed in
order to heal. Sometimes this is simply seeing the truth and

realizing that an old belief is really an illusion. The energy is healed and then released.

For example, during an energy healing session, my healer said to me, "A part of you wants to be sick." I was so appalled! I thought, "What? I want to be sick? Why on earth would I want to be sick! Are you crazy?" I was so irritated I wanted to knock her off her chair. Then she guided me back to when I was very young, around three years old. I had three brothers and three sisters, three of whom were deaf. My mom was very busy taking care of everyone. One of the ways to get my mom's attention was to be sick. So at that time I formed a belief that "Being sick brought me love and attention." Unfortunately that belief stayed in my subconscious even though I was not aware of it. Consequently, I was sick often my entire childhood, then I became very sick with CFS! Ironically as an adult, that belief was far from the truth. When I was sick all of the time I didn't get love or attention. At first I was horrified to think that I actually wanted to be sick and I felt bad for being responsible for all those years of illness. However, I came to realize that this was just one piece of the puzzle. Now at this point in the session I could see that this belief was not the truth and I could release it. This stopped my body and mind from carrying out this negative and destructive pattern.

Being Grounded

For most people, being grounded is a new concept. I first heard about it when I was driving to my first school session at the School of Energy Mastery. I was driving with another student and a teacher. We were driving from California to Wyoming. The teacher had been driving for a few hours when we pulled into the gas station. As we were getting gas, I got out and said "I can drive now if you want." And she looked at me and said, "Oh no – you are not driving – you are out of your body!" I was thinking… "Out of my body…what are you talking about? I have been driving very well for years out of my body…in fact I drove limousines for 3 years while out of my body!"

For me, it was very challenging to get grounded in my body and to stay there. Being "grounded" means being connected to your body and in touch with it. Not being grounded is when your consciousness is outside of your body. This can happen when you are uncomfortable or scared. For example, when I was in an uncomfortable situation or I felt unsafe, my pattern was to "check out" and to not be fully present. This way I didn't feel everything. I learned to do this when I was young. I didn't feel comfortable in my environment most of the time, so I was almost always "out of my body." It is similar to being on automatic pilot. You are functioning, but you are not 100% engaged and present.

For me, because I was not grounded, I was not in touch with my body and did not listen to it. I was always pushing myself and constantly overdoing it. I did not understand that I had to stop pushing myself physically and to rest and take care of myself.

Here is an exercise to ground yourself: *Sit in a chair with your spine straight. Place you feet flat on the floor shoulder width apart, hands on your thighs. Close your eyes and take a few deep breaths. Imagine a cord going from the base of your spine straight down through the floor and down into the earth. This cord connects you to the earth and keeps you grounded. Then get up and walk around staying grounded.* You can practice this anytime, anywhere.

Connecting to Yourself

What is so nice about an energy healing session is that you get in touch with your body and connected to it at a deep level. Then you can really feel what is going on. Once you have this feeling you can stay connected to your body all the time. Throughout the day you can ask yourself, "Am I pushing myself? Am I tired? Do I need to rest? Do I need to cry?" Sometimes I catch myself running around all day with so many things to accomplish no matter how tired I am. I will be getting ready to go surfing (which is a strenuous workout), and I'll close my eyes, go inside and tune into my body to see how it really feels. Sometimes my body is tired and needs to rest or do a lighter activity. So even though my mind wants to surf, I have learned to listen to what my body needs.

Connecting to Your Heart

During an Energy Healing session you also become connected to your heart so you can live your life from your heart. Most people live their life from their head, logically deciding what to do. They do what they think they should do. However, when you live your life from your heart, then you feel what you want to do. You do what makes your heart sing. Do you know what makes your heart sing? Start asking yourself and asking your heart.

Here is an exercise to connect to your heart: *On a blank sheet of paper, write down the questions: What does my heart want? What makes me happy? What am I passionate about? Then close your eyes and bring your awareness to your heart. Try to answer these questions from your heart. Imagine that your heart has a voice. For a few days keep going back to these questions to see if you have more answers.* This exercise is most powerful for me when I am by myself in nature, where there are no distractions, and it is easier to answer these questions.

Can you remember how you felt when you fell in love? You definitely don't think. You just feel love and everything is wonderful. It is actually a challenge to concentrate on your work or your studies and to be in your head, because you just want to stay in your heart and feel that love. When you are not connected to your heart, then you don't know what you really want. You've heard the saying, "Follow your heart." Well it's true! Your health and your life will change for the better when you truly follow your heart.

Beliefs

Unfortunately, when we are young and impressionable, we take on other's beliefs. These beliefs may be false, but if at the time we believe they are true, then they become our beliefs. As I mentioned in Chapter III, these beliefs and illusions are held in our body and in our subconscious; consequently, they affect the way we think and act. We may not consciously be aware of them, still, they are there - hidden in our subconscious. Energy healing as well as Meridian Tapping can reveal these hidden beliefs and release them.

Memories

We all have pictures in our subconscious of memories and traumas. Sometimes these memories are not what really happened, but how we perceived the situation. If we reacted from our wounds (which are our own issues of abandonment, jealousy, mistrust, doubt, unworthiness, etc.), then our perceptions would be distorted.

For example, growing up, I was so afraid of my father. I closed my heart and was not able to receive his love. My memory of my childhood is that he didn't love me. However, when I go back to that time I can see that he did love me very much. These memories/pictures can greatly affect our beliefs. When we go back to the time of these memories/pictures and bring God/love into these pictures, the truth is revealed and the pictures are broken and dissolved. This greatly changes our beliefs and patterns. We then become aligned with the truth.

Our Goal

Our goal is to release all of these false beliefs, negative patterns, repressed emotions, and distorted pictures. Then we can fully experience the truth, which is love.

* * *

VI

Eating Optimally

Ok…I'm not going to talk about "eating optimally" too much…but it is important to cover some basics. If you have been sick for a long time, your digestion is probably not good. Now in the beginning for the first 6 months it is most important to focus on taking the herbs in either capsules or a drink. Then your digestion will gradually improve. Eventually, you will crave more healthy foods, if you don't already eat really healthy.

Back to Basics

It is really important to NOT eat any processed foods, or foods or drinks containing any chemicals or preservatives. This includes artificial sweeteners. Our bodies are not made to break any artificial additives down. So if you want something sweet, use real sugar or buy food made with cane sugar, plain sugar or honey. Old fashioned ice cream is the best which is made out of just sugar, milk and vanilla. So read the ingredients of EVERYTHING you eat and make sure it is as simple as possible or make it yourself if you have the energy. Be aware when it says, "natural flavoring" in the ingredients, that may not be true. It is better to be able to see all the ingredients listed.

You can't drink coffee when taking the herbal program, but you can drink caffeinated tea. Just don't drink more than 4 tea bags a day. When I want a lot of caffeine I put 2 tea bags in one cup.

My Diet

I never used to be a big vegetable lover, so I have been incorporating more vegetables into my diet. Recently, I've been eating a lot of kale and I love it! I sauté garlic, onions, olive oil or coconut oil, ginger, kale and any other vegetables like broccoli, or bock choy. Sometimes I just use kale. I flavor it with Tamari sauce and spices. At the end I add coconut butter which makes it really rich. Then for protein, I mix it with Quinoa. Quinoa is a fabulous source of protein and so easy and quick to prepare. I also eat Quinoa with a little coconut milk (you could also use soy milk, almond milk or rice dream) and maple syrup for breakfast. Quinoa is really versatile. I also add it to my salads for protein. **Kale salad is easy to make and if you make a lot the night before, then it will last a couple days. You use uncooked Kale and break it up in small pieces. Put it in a big bowl. Add olive oil, lemon, pine nuts (or other nuts), red onions, and sun dried tomatoes. Put it in the refrigerator, and by the morning it will be soft.** I don't eat dairy, wheat and not much sugar. Of course sometimes I do, but most of the time I don't.

Ultimately, we should eat as much live, organic, fresh and natural food as we can. Raw food is also good for you however, if your digestion is not great...then it's hard to digest. I tried to eat all raw food a few years ago, and almost fainted one morning. My body just wasn't ready for that. If you want to eat raw foods, I suggest starting slowly. Juicing is great. Gradually adding more raw foods to your diet is the best way to go. Be patient with yourself. It may take a while for your digestion to improve.

I would ask someone who can channel your guides for you, and ask your guides what your body needs at that time. If you don't know someone who can channel your guides, I have an excellent channeler that I have used listed in the Resource section on page 114. Eventually, you want to be able to hear your own guides and guidance and be so in tune with your body that you know what it needs.

More Recipes

Chocolate Tofu Pie:

- 1 bag of either chocolate chips or carob chips (from the health food store, dairy free)
- 1 box of silk tofu firm
- Brown sugar or cane sugar – just a little – as much as you prefer

Blend the tofu in a blender so it is smooth.

Melt the chocolate chips in a frying pan on really low heat.

Add chocolate to blender and mix with tofu. Add as much sugar as needed.

Then pour evenly over either a wheat free pie crust or chopped up walnuts or almonds.

Put in the refrigerator and voila….a yummy, rich desert that is also a great snack with all the protein from the tofu and nuts if you use them for a crust!

*If you make this for others like at Thanksgiving…just don't tell them its tofu and they will never know.

Conclusion

What you eat does affect your body. So…do eat as much organic, fresh fruits, vegetables and grains as you can. And when you do want to eat comfort food, make it as healthy as possible. In the beginning, don't stress out about eating right. Just focus on taking the herbal program, then as you feel better, it will be easier to eat better.

* * *

VII

Loving Yourself

Loving yourself your self is so important in your healing process. It also affects your ability to manifest abundance and create your dream life. As I mentioned before, research has shown that, when you feel love for 5 minutes, it raises your immune system for 6 hours! In this chapter I'm going to give you some exercises that you can practice daily to love yourself more and more, ultimately loving yourself unconditionally.

Dolphin Story

It is so easy to not love yourself and not feel lovable when you are sick. I didn't realize how unlovable I felt until I swam with the dolphins in the wild on the Big Island of Hawaii. As I was swimming with them, I could feel their unconditional love and total acceptance. My heart just opened up when I was in their presence. They are so playful and loving. I swam with them for so long, following them around in big circles and watching them float up close to me and look me in the eye with that big smile that is always on their face! When I got out of the water I thought to myself, "wow they still love me and want to play with me even though I am sick!" It was then that I realized I actually had felt that way! That was such a blessing. So…consciously or unconsciously you may feel unlovable for many reasons.

You've heard the saying, "you can't love anyone else unless you love yourself". Well, that is true. Yes it is easier to love others. And for women it is natural to put everyone else's needs before ours. But now it has been revealed that we need to take care of ourselves first and then we are better equipped to take care of others. A great example of this, is when you are flying on an airplane. When there is a loss of oxygen in the cabin, the oxygen masks come down. If you have a child or someone who needs assistance, you must put on your oxygen mask first, then put on theirs, because you only have a few seconds before you pass out!

Learn how to love all parts of yourself…even the parts that are not so lovable to you. Here's an **exercise** for that:

1. Write down all the things you love about yourself (for example)
   - I love my smile
   - I love how loving I am
2. Now write down all the other things you don't really like – but write them as though you love them anyway.
   - I love how emotional I can be
   - I love all my wrinkles

Then catch yourself being critical and judging yourself and accept that part of you, then send it love. Keep doing this until you really do love yourself…all of yourself.

Attracting more Abundance, Health & Happiness

The amount of abundance, health and happiness that you allow into your life is in direct relationship with how much you love yourself. One day when I was swimming in the ocean. I was imagining living my dream life… being wealthy and doing all the things I want to do…when I had the revelation that it all depends on how much I loved myself. I was imagining having all this and then I thought, "wow, can I really live like this and have and experience all this...can I really give this to myself…do I love myself enough to receive all of this and more??? I realized that we limit what we receive with thoughts like, "oh that's too good to be true" or "I don't deserve all that, I'm sick, or I haven't earned it" etc. etc. That's not true. We do deserve everything. There is no limit to what we can do or have, except our own limits. So you see, loving yourself is also related to how much abundance you allow in.

Do you have any regrets, guilt, or shame about past mistakes? Maybe subconsciously you are beating yourself up for doing this or not doing that. If there is a yes to any of this, stop now and let's do a quick exercise, or write it down on a piece of paper to do later.

Exercise: To release guilt and shame from your past

- *Sit comfortably. Close your eyes. Take a few deep breaths.*
- *Imagine there is a bubble in front of you with a big magnet in the middle*
- *Now imagine and intend that all the shame and guilt from your past and present is drawn out from your body and into this bubble*
- *Take a deep breath*
- *Now call back all of your power from this bubble*
- *Imagine your power coming back into your body*
- *Now imagine you are popping that bubble in front of you and all that shame and guilt is being transmuted into the light*
- *Take a deep breath*

* You can also do Meridian Tapping (EFT) with these emotions.

You can do this bubble exercise with other issues, feelings, or memories you want to release or take your power back from. After you have done it once, you will be able to keep your eyes closed and not have to read the instructions.

Remember that we are all here to learn from our mistakes. So keep loving yourself and don't worry if you don't do something right. You are loved and lovable just the way you are...really!!!

More Exercises:

- *Twice a day – ask your self, "what's the most loving thing I could do for myself right now?" Then feel in your body to get an answer. It could be to: take a nap, drink some water, eat something, meditate, go for a walk, sit outside, be in nature, whatever it is for you.*

Another Exercise: Do this 2-4 times a day

- *Put your hand over your heart*
- *Imagine breath coming in and out through your heart*
- *On the breath in bring love, compassion and ease in*
- *Exhale normally*
- *Breath this way 4-5 times*

Similar Exercise:

- *Sit comfortably*
- *Close your eyes*
- *Bring attention to your heart*
- *Breath in love*
- *Feel the love expand into your body and every cell*
- *Fill your entire body with love, even parts that feel tense*
- *Say out loud to yourself, "I love me, I love myself"*
- *Sit in this tingly loving feeling as long as you like*

The more you do these exercises, the more you will love yourself, heal yourself and radiate your love and light. Give compassion to the parts of you that you feel are unlovable. Love heals everything.

Conclusion

Love yourself, love one another, love, love, love. See love in EVERYTING. When fear comes up, let it go and give it to God and the Angels and choose love in that moment. Ask to be shown the love – "Where is the love?" "Show me the love." Put an imaginary filter over your eyes or imaginary glasses that filter all the fear and negativity. So you only see the LOVE in EVERYTHING. Instead of "rose colored" glasses, you can wear "love filtered" glasses and see everything through love with love. Being in the love and staying connected to the love is what keeps you in alignment with God, your higher self and your soul. Accept where you are. Be compassionate with yourself, and love yourself unconditionally.

✳ ✳ ✳

VIII

Connecting to God & Your Higher Self

Connecting to God and your higher self is a very important key to healing and living in radiant health and happiness. As I mentioned earlier, I was so angry with God for letting me suffer and be sick for so many years. I didn't realize that I cut off my connection to God/Source. For so many years of being sick, I felt so alone and unsupported. It was during my first energy healing session, when I was re-connected with God, and could really feel his love and support, that my health started to improve. Then I had the strength, trust and courage to keep fighting and heal.

We are always connected to God, the Angels, the Universe and our higher self at a deep level. However, we can lose that or feel like we have lost that connection when we experience fear, anger, sadness, guilt, or shame. At every moment there is a choice of either love or fear. If we stay in the love, we stay connected and aligned to our higher self and God. If we go into fear or other emotions related to fear, we don't feel that connection.

Some of you reading this may have never really experienced this connection. If so, a healer or I can help you feel this connection with God. I have listed a few healers in the referral section at the end. Then when you quiet your mind and connect more often, it will get easier and quicker to connect.

Here is a message I channeled from the Angels for you:

Dear ones know that you are not alone. We are always with you and here for you. Many of you feel lost and abandoned, scared and weak because you have lost your connection. Rather you feel like you have lost your connection. But dear ones, you can never lose that connection. It is always there, you just get lost and don't feel it or trust that it is indeed there. Quieting the mind helps. Go inside, tone, connect to your higher self and soul regularly, and eventually you will always feel connected.

The unlimited love from God, the Angels, and the Universe feeds you. Don't feel bad about feeling disconnected. It is easy to do and done by most of your planet you see – but now is the time to connect again and remember who you are. Remember what you came here to do. Wake up – the time is now to shed the old baggage, excuses, doubts, fears, generalizations, judgments, assumptions, false beliefs, illusions and see the light. See the truth and be the truth.

Being sick is the old paradigm and matrix. There is no need for it anymore. There are no more reasons to hide dear ones. You will be seen and heard, and it is safe for you to come out of hiding!

Remember, there is no right or wrong. Everything is a choice. You can be attached to your labels of being sick and attached to any kind of identity you have chosen to give your power to. The truth is – you can do and be whatever you desire. It is a matter of re-conditioning your mind and allowing your true self to come out.

Some emotions and traumas are so powerful that you have become stuck in "pause" mode with a label of being sick or having CFS or whatever it is. It is really not about the label or the illness, it is about taking care of yourself, loving and honoring yourself. Believe that anything is possible and if you are ready to heal…then the help will come – like this book – and the herbal program to normalize your polarity.

Hearing Your Own Guidance

Ultimately, you want to be able to hear your own guidance and be able to feel what your body needs. This is the same as following your intuition. You know that feeling you get when you are driving and you sense that you should go a certain way, then find out later, there was a bad accident on the road you usually take? That gut feeling and sensation is your intuition. In the beginning of your healing process or wherever you are on your healing journey, it is helpful to get guidance and support from healers, and experts, then eventually be able to hear your own guidance.

Recently I took an online course on channeling at www.lightworker.com. It was called spiritual communication. They say that everyone on the planet will be doing this someday. We all have the ability to hear our own guidance and to receive messages from God, and the Angels and other light beings. Many of us are born doing this naturally, then we get programmed to shut it off.

Tips for hearing your own guidance:

- Being in nature is a great way to connect to God and your higher self. I like to sit in a beach chair with a pen and paper and write down messages I receive.
- Being by water is also inspiring and can stimulate that flow.
- To prepare yourself to channel or connect, sit in a chair with your left leg crossed over your right knee. Put your right hand on your left ankle, and put your left hand on your right upper arm just below your shoulder. Take a few deep breaths. This can clear your energy and open up your channel to receive messages.
- Meditation of course is excellent to get centered and quiet your mind so you can hear your guidance.

Meditating to Connect to Your Higher Self

Meditation is a great way to connect to your higher self, which is part of your heart, your soul, and your spirit. Your higher self is also connected to God, and the unlimited knowledge of the universe. This is where your intuition comes from. It is a powerful inner wisdom that can be heard when you are tuned into it or your mind is quiet enough to hear it. It is possible to always be connected to it. So during meditation you can ask yourself questions such as, "What does my heart want? What should I do about this situation? What is for my highest good?" When your mind is quiet, you will hear a response, feel a response, get a picture, or just have a knowing. In the beginning you may wonder if the message you are getting is from your higher self, from God, or it's your voice. After a while you will be able to know. The more you listen to your higher self (your intuition) the more familiar you will become with it.

Our higher self or sometimes called our true self - is always peaceful, joyous, in the love, strong, and knowing. You can meditate with the intention to be aligned with your higher self. Throughout the day many things can cause you to fall out of this alignment. For example, someone may say something that hurts you. Next thing you know - you feel hurt and weak and not your strong and happy self. This is when you can close your eyes and imagine that you are connected and aligned with your higher self. Now throughout the day - whenever I feel like I am out of alignment, I close my eyes, take a few breaths and imagine that I am connected to my higher self, God, love and peace. The more I do this - the easier it gets and the faster I regain my alignment. I also achieve this by toning. Toning centers me within one minute. *To tone, simply close your eyes, take a deep breath, and when you exhale keep your mouth closed and make a sound - similar to humming.* The sound you are making brings your awareness inside.

Exercise:

Sit quietly. Close your eyes. Take a couple deep breaths, Relax. Call on Arch Angel Michael, Jesus, Buddha, your Guardian Angel, whomever you wish, and ask them to come into your heart. Imagine you are meeting them in a sacred chamber in your heart. Imagine they are in front of you. Look at them and ask them a question. Wait quietly for an answer. Ask as many questions as you wish. You can write the answers down. For me, I receive messages by writing them down. Some people get pictures, hear a voice, feel something, or get a knowing.

We all have guardian angels. When I was getting a massage on the Big Island a few years ago, I arrived about 10 minutes late. Then I had to use the rest room so I said, "I'm sorry I'm late, and now I have to use the rest room." The masseuse replied, "Oh don't worry dear, you guardian angels haven't arrived yet." I had never heard that before, but it really resonated with me and solidified my belief in guardian angels.

Another Channeling for you:

Dear ones remember who you are…you are pure light, love, the essence of all that is. As you awaken from your sleep be kind to yourself and others. Be who you came here to be. Give up all your pain and suffering to be transmuted into the light. You are safe. You are loved. You are appreciated. All is well and as it should be. Listen to your heart. Listen to each other. Love yourself and honor yourself.

You are always connected at a deep level. It is at this deep level that you will find your higher self, your guidance and all the answers you seek. Great wisdom is within you dear ones. Close your eyes, breathe deeply, and relax. Bring your awareness deep into your body into your heart, your sacred heart, which is where your infinite love, light and wisdom reside. The more you connect to this part of you, the easier it becomes. Throughout the day you can you can connect to this sanctuary of peace, love and bliss whenever you want wherever you are. Let this love, light, peace and bliss permeate out of your being and into the world. Let this loving peaceful energy go into everything you do and think. Know that this peace, love, light and bliss is available to all of you all the time.

Conclusion

It is this love and light from God and the Angels that give you the support and courage to heal and live a healthy and happy life. The beautiful thing about this love and light is that it is available to all of you and can never be taken away. So even if you don't currently have great health, or don't have financial abundance, whatever your situation is…you still have this amazing connection to God and the Angels to access and feel this radiant love and light, which is truly healing. The more you bask in this pure love and light…the quicker you will heal and attain radiant health and happiness.

* * *

IX

THE POWER OF YOUR MIND

As you can see by now from all that you have read so far...your mind is extremely powerful! Your mind is your biggest tool for healing. Your thoughts have the power to affect your body physiologically. Ester Hicks has been channeling information from "Abraham" for many years now about the Law of Attraction. Abraham states that, "Your body is a reflection of the balance of your thoughts." Therefore, it is really important to be aware of your thoughts. Fortunately, when your polarity is normalized, you will be thinking clearly, and it will be easier to monitor your thoughts. The Law of Attraction states that *you attract what you think about*. So, your thoughts are creating your reality.

The Law of Attraction

People need to give themselves permission to heal and be happy and yes...to have whatever it is that they want. The power of the Law of Attraction is so immense. Once you have cleared your limiting beliefs and patterns, anything is possible! All you have to do is imagine what you want, visualize you are having it or doing it, really believe and know that it is possible, then allow it to come to you in any form. You should do this often because your body does not differentiate whether what you are thinking about is real or imaginary. By doing this you are re-programming your body and mind to be healthy and strong again, and it feels so good! I used to do this often. I would imagine I was skiing down a wide ski slope, carving big arching giant slalom turns. I would remember exactly what it felt like to have really strong legs and to be able to ski so powerfully.

So go ahead and imagine that you are living your ideal life with endless energy and the ability to do whatever you want. As I mentioned, for me it was skiing down the mountain so effortlessly with the fresh, crisp air caressing my face. Gliding so smoothly through the trees it was as if I was flying through the forest with the sunlight glistening on the snow and sparkling like diamonds. What a tremendous exhilaration this is! Because I am such a good skier, I can ski down anything which results in me feeling like I can do anything and accomplish anything in life.

Now imagine running down the street or on the beach or a trail through the woods and really tune into the feeling of your body being in such great shape that it is effortless and exhilarating. Imagine whatever it is that you love to do that makes you feel strong and healthy. It could even be riding in a speed boat or sailboat with the air brushing by and the exhilaration of gliding on the water.

The Steps to Manifesting your Desires

Ask for what you desire and be very specific. What is the essence of what you desire? What will it feel like when you receive it?

Imagine already having it and how it will make you feel. Imagine every detail. How does it look? What do you smell? What do you hear? What are you feeling?

Allow what you desire to come into your life is the final and most important step. I have found that loving yourself is in direct correlation with being able to allow what you desire into your life. The more you love yourself and feel worthy...the more you are able to receive and allow into your life.

Now when I ask the universe for something I ask myself, "Do I love myself enough to give this to me, and to allow this gift into my life now?" You may be surprised at what your response is, especially if it is something that you are asking for to come in a way that is not normal or part of the normal way. For example, asking for a large some of money and assuming it can only come by working at a certain job or doing the normal service in order to receive such an amount. Another key point is to release your desires to God and the Universe so that they can come in any form.

For many of us we are conditioned as children to limit what we can have and definitely limit the way in which we receive things. Some people are taught not to take anything for free, or that you must work hard for something, and this makes it harder for people to receive gifts, help or support. Then when you are asking for something, you have all these limiting conditions about how to receive it. Are you are even worthy or deserving etc.? These can be hidden in your subconscious like I spoke about earlier in Chapter III (Unconscious Emotions & Beliefs). To reveal some of these limiting beliefs, you can *sit down. Close your eyes. Take a few deep breaths. Be still, and ask yourself if you deserve this desire or what you feel about receiving this desire…and see what comes up.*

For example, with me right now as I'm writing this book…I don't have an agent or publisher yet. So I occasionally, ask myself, "Can I really do this? Can I really get an agent and a publisher and have people read it all over the world?" Then I feel how passionate I am about this and get in touch with the knowing I have deep down inside that this is my path and then I can say to myself, "Yes of course I am doing this." Then I also open up to other ways of getting this book out all over the world. So also be sure to focus on the end result as there may be many different ways to achieve your desired outcome. "I am publishing my book and helping people all over the world!" Then I stay in this feeling and the more I connect with this feeling and knowing, the less the doubts come up. Doubts are normal, we all have them.

The Law of Attraction is about focusing only on what you want and not on your current reality. Keep focusing only on what you want your life to be and how it will feel. This can be feeling peace, financial security, radiant health, love, etc. whatever it is that you desire. This can be challenging because it is so natural for us to focus on and think about what we have now or don't have or on what we don't want. Like, "I don't want to be poor, I don't want to live in this small condo I'm living in," etc. So don't ask from your current state of lack or disappointment, ask from the state that you are already living abundantly. For example: "I am grateful for the money I have now and I'm ready for more and more money to come to me." Think and speak in positive sentences. Always ask for what you want in the positive. For example: don't say, "I intend that I have more money so that I am not stressed," Say, "I intend that I have more money so that I am relaxed and at peace." In fact the more you think about all the positive reasons you want your desire the more your body begins to feel it as if it has already happened, then your vibration will eventually attract it to you.

      I also like to say, "I am so happy and grateful now that I am making at least $5,000 a month." Or, "I'm so happy and grateful now that I am arriving at the hotel for my appointment at 10:00am easily and effortlessly." Many times I do this when I am running late. I imagine pulling into my destination and seeing 10:00am on the clock in my car. It works every time! For more information, I suggest reading and or listening to Abram – Hicks material on the Law of Attraction. They have books, CDs, DVDs and workshops. Their website is: www.abraham-hicks.com

Conclusion

Your mind is powerful. Fortunately, you can control it! Now with all the tools you have learned to re-program your mind and body, you are ready to use the Law of Attraction and consciously create radiant health and happiness.

* * *

In Summary

The Keys to Attain Radiant Health & Happiness

- Normalize your polarity with the Herbal Program 4-6 months.

- When your polarity is normalized, your mind will be clear so you can identify and release unconscious limiting emotions, beliefs and patterns with Tapping, Hypnotherapy, or Angel Therapy.

- Re-program the way your body reacts to stress with Tapping and meditation.

- Release the label of "Chronic Fatigue Syndrome" or whatever illness or condition you have and take your power back – as it is really just the name of a condition you are currently experiencing. It has no power over you.

- Take responsibility for your healing and your life. Release your "victim" mentality and empower yourself. Know that you create your own reality.

- Strengthen your connection with God, the Angels and your higher self and follow your own guidance.

- Monitor your thoughts and only think about the way you want your life to be and how you want to feel.

- Use the Law of Attraction to consciously create Radiant Health and Happiness.

May you attain Radiant Health & Happiness!

Love and Blessings,

Margo

RESOURCES

Margo Nagy

Coach for Healing CFS and Certified Reiki Practitioner

www.polaritybalancing.net

(808)652-9599

Keith Smith

Master Herbalist

(Created the Herbal Program to un-reverse your polarity)

The Herb Shop

Escondido, Ca

www.keithrsmith.com

(760)489-6889

Nelly Coneway

Hypnotherapist and Angel Therapy Practitioner

(Can channel your guides and Angels)

www.happyyogi.net

(808)212-8252

Lynda Farr

Certified Level II (EFT) Emotional Freedom Technique Practitioner

www.stresslessprograms.com

(414)315-2021

Carol Conley, MFT

Marriage and Family Therapist

(Uses Tapping (EFT) in her practice)

(808)635-2597

ABOUT THE AUTHOR

At age 19, Margo Nagy was a world class athlete aspiring to be on the US Ski Team when she was diagnosed with Chronic Fatigue Syndrome (CFS). For the next 26 years of her life, she struggled with paralyzing fatigue, depression, insomnia, brain fog, and almost died.

Margo has researched and personally experienced most healing modalities, making her an expert in the field of healing. After successfully recovering from Chronic Fatigue Syndrome, she is living proof that one can heal from CFS and Depression, to achieve radiant health and happiness. Because of this experience, she is able to give the kind of support, understanding, empowerment, guidance, inspiration and hope that only a CFS survivor can give.

Margo is a graduate of the School of Energy Mastery where she studied Energy Healing and learned the importance of healing the body, mind and spirit. She is a certified Reiki Practitioner, and holds a BA in International Business from San Diego State University.

Currently, Margo offers coaching for people with CFS or other chronic illnesses. Her website is www.polaritybalancing.net which includes her Blog and a video about Chronic Reversed Polarity on YouTube.

Margo is passionate, charismatic, funny and inspirational. Her radiant health and enthusiasm is felt by everyone who comes in contact with her. Today she surfs, skis, hikes, does yoga and swims in the oceans of her Kauai home. Her mission is to help others heal while raising the planet's consciousness and vibration.

What I am going to do when I get better:

- _____

- _____

- _____

- _____

- _____

- _____

- _____

- _____

- _____

- _____

What does my heart desire?

- _____
- _____
- _____
- _____
- _____
- _____
- _____
- _____
- _____
- _____

How can I love and nourish myself?

- _____
- _____
- _____
- _____
- _____
- _____
- _____
- _____
- _____
- _____

What are my limiting beliefs and patterns:

- _____
- _____
- _____
- _____
- _____
- _____
- _____
- _____
- _____
- _____

What do I need to heal and release (with tapping):

- _____
- _____
- _____
- _____
- _____
- _____
- _____
- _____
- _____
- _____

My desired story: (How I desire my life to be – written in present tense)

_____

_____

_____

_____

_____

_____

_____

_____

_____

What I am grateful for:

- _____
- _____
- _____
- _____
- _____
- _____
- _____
- _____
- _____
- _____
- _____
- _____
- _____
- _____

DISCLAIMER

The information in this book is not intended to diagnose, treat, or cure any disease or psychological disorder. This book does not guarantee the cure for any illness, or condition. The author makes no warranty or guarantee for the cure of any illness or condition. While all materials and references to other resources are given in good faith, the accuracy, validity, effectiveness or usefulness of any information in this book cannot be guaranteed. The author accepts no responsibility or liability whatsoever for the use or misuse of the information contained in this book, including links to other resources.